Further Reflections

From Common Ground

Cultural Awareness in Healthcare

Beth Lincoln, MSN, RN

with narratives by Cody Gillette Kirkham

Copyright 2017

Printed in the United States
ISBN-13: 978-1540772473
ISBN-10: 1540772470

For more information visit our website Celemonde!
www.celemonde.com

Cover design: Jon Dodge

Dedication

*To the voices of patients and families
that call us to tell their story*

Nowhere is globalization more evident than in the healthcare industry. Patients and healthcare professionals need to work together as partners in care. In addressing this need, Beth Lincoln has written a remarkable follow up to her first edition of *Reflections from Common Ground*. In this informative and thought-provoking second edition, Lincoln again offers vignettes which bring the chapters to life – we see ourselves, our families, friends, neighbors, and patients in these poignant stories. In *Further Reflections from Common Ground*, Lincoln presents sensitive issues related to marginalized cultural groups who need their stories to be told. She expertly guides the reader through a maze of misunderstandings, biases, expectations, and misperceptions to common ground.

Beth Desaretz Chiatti, PhD, RN, CTN-B, CSN
Assistant Clinical Professor
Drexel University, Philadelphia, PA

A powerful call to take account of our beliefs, values, and biases. In *Further Reflections from Common Ground,* Lincoln inspires, challenges, and motivates us to provide culturally sensitive and competent care to all patients, especially those who have felt marginalized, misunderstood or "mistreated" by the healthcare system. Lincoln encourages us to acknowledge the unique talents that colleagues bring to the table, and to work together to provide equitable health care. A must read for all who work in health care. You will return to your work community with new eyes and appreciation.

Dee McFarland M.Ed
Education Consultant - Cultural Awareness & Competence

My staff used first book, *Reflections from Common Ground: Cultural Awareness in Healthcare,* as a reference on a number of occasions, so I see the second book as a great follow-up to be used in a similar fashion. Both books help us look honestly at ourselves and our prejudices. Until we do that, we can't, truly, be open to someone else's world view – to go beyond mere tolerance.

Jan Darter RN
Maternity Manager
St Helena, CA

...the common eye sees only the outside of things,
and judges by that,
but the seeing eye pierces through
and reads the heart and the soul,
finding there capacities
which the outside didn't indicate or promise, and
which the other kind couldn't detect.

Mark Twain
Personal Recollections of Joan of Arc

Table of Contents

Dedication
Peer Review
Chapters
1. Perception is not always Reality 1
2. History . . . We All Have a Story 5
3. Growing More Diverse . . . Trends Over Time 19
4. It's Time to Have the Conversation 31
5. Access to Care . . . What Gets in the Way? 43
6. Finding Common Ground   63
7. Ancient Wisdom . . . Modern Medicine. 79
8. Elsa's Story . . . Can you see me? Emergency Preparedness - The Deaf Community . . . 97
9. Jeremiah's Story . . . Shut up & Listen Urgent Care - Homeless Youth 113
10. Ev's story . . I am not going back! Cancer - The Lesbian Community 127
11. Suki's Story When Home Remedies May Not Be Enough Home Safety - Amish 143
12. Harjit's Story . . . Please Let Me Go . . . A Good Death End of Life - Hindu 157
13. Shin's Story . . . Can't you control your child! Autism & the Korean Family 171
14. Liliya's Story . . . It's not my job . . . It's yours! Diabetes & the Russian Immigrant . . .185
15. Fusaye's Story . . . Meeting Expectations? Suicide & the Japanese Family. 199
16. Theodora & Melina's Story . . . Exhaustion! Care Givers & the Greek Family. 217
17. Conchita's Story - Too much weight? Obesity & Cuban Family 233
18. Carlito's Story . . . I can't breath! Asthma - Prison - Puerto Rican 247
19. Mauve's Story . . . Creating the Illusion - Alcoholism & the Irish Family 263
20. Sammy's Story . . . Belonging Gangs - Youth 279
21. Diversity & Inclusion . . . The Best of All Worlds 293
22. Closing Thoughts. 307

Appendix. 311
Glossary 323
Index 327
Footnotes 332
About the Author 342

Perception is not always Reality

1

Even though Marina and Ivan try hard not to show it, Liliya knows they resent her presence in their five hundred square foot apartment. She should have stayed in Vladivostok instead of following her daughter. Liliya had a good job at home---she can never think of Napa as "home"---and she really enjoyed managing the personnel office at the credit union where she worked six days a week. She does love telling people what to do, which job might capitalize on their strengths, which salary would be out of the question. She had no trouble in Russia being forthright. As she enters the Bank of the West, trying once more for even a menial position, Liliya adjusts her sling-back shoes, pushes her recently dyed hair behind her ears, and extends a hand. The office manager is expecting her. There is a sizable Russian population in the upper valley here, and Carol is hoping that Liliya will be like Lara in Dr. Zhivago; it is obvious that she is not. Liliya is overweight and overly forward, too much in several regards if appearances are to be believed. "So I come for the job behind the table in your bank. I am head of office in Russia. I work with people. How much you pay for job like that?"

The demographics have changed dramatically in the United States over the past half century. The once predominant white community is now trending toward a more multi-ethnic population. New immigrants, such as Liliya, come to reunite with their families. Others are seeking a better life with more opportunity. Each person brings their cultural beliefs and values about health and care. Expectations of a healthcare system reflective of their country of origin may be not be realized.

Navigating the U.S. healthcare system adds to their unease and frustration. In Chapter 14 we meet Liliya, an elderly Russian immigrant with diabetes. She came from Russia to live with her daughter and family in the United States. Her limited English skills interfere with the ability to communicate her healthcare needs. She is most annoyed by her physician's adamancy that she be an active participant in the management of her diabetes. Diabetic self-management, from her perspective, is not the Russian way. In Russia she is not expected to monitor her blood sugars or record her dietary intake. Rather, she is expected to attend monthly visits to the sanitarium for a blood test and a physical exam. As with many new immigrants, she holds a strong connection to the 'Russia way' of healthcare. Understanding her perspective may be challenging to her healthcare professional (HCP). However, it is essential to consider her cultural beliefs, values and health practices when planning her care. While, assimilation and adjustment are the challenge for Liliya, cultural awareness, sensitivity and competency are the challenge for us.

Think about your clinical setting. What is the demographic make-up of your patient population? In the past eighteen months, have you received inservice education on the importance of providing culturally competent care to the people you serve? Techniques on communicating across cultures? End of life care from a cultural perspective? These subjects and more provide the building blocks and pathways for HCPs to find common ground, establish patient rapport, and provide culturally sensitive and competent healthcare. The result – we avert misunderstandings and assure good health outcomes.

Further Reflections From Common Ground features rarely mentioned groups such as prisoners, Deaf community, homeless youth, street gangs and the Lesbian-Gay-Bisexual-Transgender community. In addition, sensitive subject matter such as suicide, autism, caregiver burnout, emergency preparedness and obesity are addressed from an ethnic perspective. Reflective exercises, placed strategically throughout the book, provide the reader an opportunity to consider similarities and differences with patients/families. Discovering common ground lays the foundation from which to build rapport and establish trust. Yes, it is a challenge for each person involved in this discussion – HCP and patient/family. Displaying a genuine interest in a patient's response to health and illness questions demonstrates an interest in their perspective. This leads to clarity, insight and quality healthcare.

My Challenge to you . . .

Be the voice, a strong, unrelenting voice, that encourages others around you to step up and embrace the benefits of delivering culturally sensitive and competent care. Watch for signs of increased satisfaction on your patients faces and the improved health outcomes that follow.

Now consider taking this same approach with your colleagues and administrators.

Your story and those of your colleagues are unique. As a result, every healthcare professional provides an extraordinary insight into the constructs of culturally competent care. Recognizing and valuing diverse viewpoints leads to an inclusive environment that acknowledges the individual's gifts and talents. A respectful and appreciative interaction is guaranteed to make a positive difference.

Enjoy the journey!

History . . . We All Have a Story | 2

Telling your story . . .

> *Reflective Exercise: Your Story . . .*
> 1. *When did your ancestors first come to America?*
> 2. *Or were they already here?*
> 3. *Why did they come?*
> 4. *How is your story similar to your colleagues & your patients?*

Speaking in his native Pomo language, a recent conference speaker explained that his grandfather told him "Your life is your story . . . tell your story." Whatever our native language, we all have a story to tell: in sharing our story, we gain insights into our history and those who came before us. Our histories, our stories, shape who we are and influence how we see and interpret our world.

Recently a young woman shared that she had fled Cambodia and spent four years in a refugee camp in Thailand before immigrating to the United States. Her colleagues never knew that piece of her history. It now provides perspective, a way of seeing her with new understanding. Now transfer this process to your patients and colleagues. How is their story similar to yours? How is it different? Where do you find common ground?

In this chapter we will look at history and the effect it may have on healthcare decisions. For some the reason to seek, or not seek, healthcare may be based on previous encounters by family members or a long standing history of mistrust of the healthcare system. Although these incidents may have happened many years in the past, it is in sharing of stories that one formulates beliefs, values, and biases about healthcare and healthcare providers.

Our story begins . . .

. . . with those who were here in America before the immigration of peoples from Europe and Asia. It begins with the Native Americans, who on the shores of the Atlantic Ocean stood watching the first white settlers arrive in this, their country. Until that time, there were, according to Charles Mann author of *1491: New Revelations about Americas before Columbus,* over 90 million Indians living on 400 million acres.[1] Their advanced level of farming, hunting and gathering had sustained them over thousands of years. It was a thriving community of peoples across the Americas, North and South. The first of many treaties with the Native American population began in the early 1800s when then Major General Andrew Jackson defeated the Creeks in what is now the state of Alabama. Over twenty million acres of tribal land was seized in the 1814 treaty. The desire by Americans to establish a solid economic base, along with the disregard for the native people currently inhabiting the land, continued this process for the next one hundred years.

Economics seems to always be at the forefront of immigration to the Americas. The early 17th century saw increased immigration from England, people seeking a better life for themselves and their families. The 1700s and 1800s brought immigrants all seeking work with the plan to send money home. They came from Italy, Germany, Ireland, Asia and South America. For many the intent was to return to their homeland, but less than half realized that dream. Other emigrations stemmed from wars, famines, and reunification. Forced immigration (slavery) added to the socioeconomic status of the plantation owner, but did nothing for that of the slave. Forced migration, the movement of people to a land inconsistent with their life style, affected most of the Native Americans who had not already been killed by guns or germs. Immigration by white settlers, unfortunately, brought disharmony and distrust.

Troubled times leads to Emigration

England

Following King Henry VIII's establishment of the Anglican church, Protestants and Catholics alike were subject to shunning by neighbors, and were also fined and occasionally jailed by the government. Some Protestants took the Reformation as an opportunity to go one step further and "purify" the Anglican church. They called themselves Puritans and believed that they did not need an intermediary (priest), but could talk to God on their own. This created a religious tumult in England. The North American colonies probably seemed like an answer to prayer: the possibility of religious freedom. In 1620 the Pilgrims, as they came to be known, sailed on the Mayflower for the new colonies.

The 17th century focused on the establishment of colonies. During this time the economy in England was unstable, and inflation led to poverty, making it next to impossible for the poor to meet even their basic needs. For many, the opportunity to leave for the new colonies was the answer. By the mid-1600s over 30,000 people had left for the new colonies. King James 1 viewed this as a win-win for England: an outlet for surplus population and input of material for their expansive industry.

As time went on, there was a greater sense of establishment in this new country with a growing desire to separate from England's rule. What followed was the Declaration of Independence in 1776. It is interesting to note that it was not until 1787 that the term immigrant was used. The term differentiated between colonists, who saw themselves as the established society, and those *foreigners* who arrived after the country's laws, customs, language, and constitution were formed. This may have been done in response to Thomas Malthus' published *Essay on Principles of Population* in 1789. It stated that England was fast running out of food production and predicted that if nothing changed, starvation would result. A surge of immigrants to America followed. Wars and famine were another reason for migration

China

In China the Opium Wars involving England (1836) and France (1846), created a very difficult situation. Because the wars decimated the land, agriculture was slow to recover and famine was the order of the day. Since there was not enough food to sustain families, many Chinese men immigrated to America to work on the railroads, in the gold mines, in agriculture, and in factories. Sending money home and repaying the merchant

who had brought them to the United States forced them to work at low wages. While many Chinese were successful and thrived, residents of the United States saw this as a threat to their livelihood. Chinese communities formed as a source of support, but stories of prostitution, gambling, and opium dens sparked the sentiment that admitting Chinese to the United States lowered the cultural and moral standards of American society (U.S. Department of State). Anti-Chinese sentiment rose and pursuant to a downturn in the economy, legislation was passed to bar immigration from China. That 1882 law, known as The Chinese Exclusion Act of 1882, was renewed in 1892 and again in 1902. It was not repealed until 1943.

Ireland

Poor economic conditions and famine played a key role in the Irish coming to American as well. Farmers in Ireland rarely owned the land, but rather rented it from landowners living in England. The cost of running the farm, however, left little money with which to support themselves and their families. Emigration to America began in the early 1800s and escalated following the potato famines of 1845 and 1846. One fourth of the population emigrated to the United States. On a recent trip to Ireland, our tour guide, Sean O'Malley, shared his family history with us. "The only time I ever heard my great grandfather talk about the great famine was during a family celebration. He recalled the people who left. It was the thought at that time that when someone left they would never be mentioned again. It was as if they had died." You could hear the sadness in Sean's voice as he told his story.

Italy and Germany

With increased taxation and low wages in Italy in 1870, many people emigrated to the United States. The intention was to make money and then return home. Many were not able to fulfill their dream; however, emigration to the U.S. continued from many European countries. It is noted that between 1820 and 1920, 4,400,000 immigrated from Ireland, 5,500,000 from Germany and 4,190,000 from Italy. Most came for the same reasons: looking for economic stability and a better life for themselves and their families. (Brunner 1997).

Mexico

Following the Mexican American War of 1848, those living in the southwestern area of the country, which was ceded to the United States by Mexico, were given U.S. citizenship with all the rights and privileges of others already living in the state. The Treaty of Guadalupe Hidalgo promised citizenship, freedom of religion and language, and maintenance of their lands. The Mexicans who lived in the southwest were subject to discrimination and social injustice following the war. Loss of both property and rights followed as well (McGoldrick 2005). Socioeconomic stability and labor needs have continued to play an integral part in the migration from Mexico to the United States. Borders, being permeable and allowing for flow back and forth, met the needs of both countries. In the mid-1800s laborers were provided by Mexico to work on the railroad and in agriculture thus proving a source of income for the Mexicans and a source of revenue for their country. This win-win relationship continued into the early 1900s, until there was a sudden downturn in the economy: the Great Depression. All immigration stopped. It was not until there was a labor shortage during World War II that the borders reopened. The Bracero program, instituted in 1942 by the United States and the Mexican government, allowed Mexican men to work in the U.S. fields for low wages. The Bracero program caused resentment with the farms workers. Cesar Chavez initiated the Farm Workers Union to support those working in agriculture with a just wage and better living conditions. The Bracero Program ended in 1964 due to pressure from the union.

The needs of individuals, regardless of their countries of origin, played a significant role in the search for stability and economic security for themselves and their families. When there is a socioeconomic downturn, there may be a perception that immigrants are taking away jobs by working for low wages. The facts do not always back up that notion. Yet, when there is a threat to economic wellbeing, fear, anger, and uncertainty loom.

Forced immigration . . . Slavery

Economics. The reasons for slavery may be many, but the bottom line was economic. Slaves are laborers who are owned: laborers who are told what to do, laborers who are told how to live. African slaves in the U.S. prior to 1865 had no rights and were considered less than whole people. They were counted as 3/5 of a person in the census report (U.S. Constitution, 1787). It is said that between three and twenty-four million slaves were brought to the United States. It does remain a fact that slavery existed for over three hundred years in this country. Families were separated. Men, women, and children were bought and sold. Living conditions were well below standard. Treatment of, and punishment for, perceived "crimes" was harsh. Slavery is a part of our story: it continues to influence us.

Not until the conclusion of the U.S. Civil War was slavery abolished. The passage of the 13th, 14th, and 15th amendments, abolished slavery and established the right of citizenship, which included the right to own land and serve on a jury. Unfortunately "Jim Crowe" laws, anti-African legislation followed these constitutional amendments, continuing to affect the former slaves' ability to realize their constitutional rights. It would be years later with the passage of the 1964 Civil Rights Act and the 1965 Voting Rights Act, that the laws established one hundred years earlier would actually take effect and become reality.

Forced migration . . . & its effects

The recent PBS documentary, *Our National Parks* (2009), emphasized that much of the the land in parks such as Yosemite, Yellowstone, Zion, and the Grand Canyon had been home to the native population for thousands of years. Displacement of Native Americans through forced migration from the "familiar" to unfamiliar land (which came to be known as reservations) changed their way of life. The *Indian Removal Act of 1830* authorized the federal government to negotiate treaties with Indian nations, exchanging their current homeland for land in the West. After treaties had been signed some of the Indians left while others remained. In 1827, the Cherokee Nation adopted a written constitution declaring itself a sovereign nation legally capable of ceding their own land. The state of Georgia (where they resided) did not recognize that sovereignty. In 1831 the Cherokee nation took its case to the Supreme Court, and while winning its appeal initially, had its decision revoked later. Forced migration occurred throughout the 1830s from the *Trail of Tears* of the Cherokee Nation to Oklahoma, to "forced march" of the Piautes from Owens Valley to Fort Tejon in California. In each case, thousands of persons perished due to lack of food, disease, and harsh conditions. Millions of acres were lost, but more than that, lost was the land that had been home for hundreds of years.

The Bureau of Indian Affairs formed in 1824. Responsible for the management of millions of acres of land "held in trust by the United States for the American Indians," the Bureau provided Indian health and socials services in exchange for the land and natural resources. In 1978 Public Law 95-341 was enacted. The law stated "it shall be the policy of the United States to protect and preserve for American Indians their inherent right of freedom to believe, express and exercise the traditional religions of the American Indian, Eskimo, Aleut and Native Hawaiian, including but not limited to access to sites, use and possession of sacred objects and the freedom to worship through ceremonials and traditional sites." (U.S. Department of the Interior). Prior to this, American Indians did not have access to a number of sacred sites situated on federal lands such as national parks.

Another attempt to change the life of the Native American was the formation of the Carlisle Indian Schools in 1879. Started by Richard Henry Pratt whose adage was "kill the Indian, save the man," the schools ensured that children who attended were prohibited from speaking their tribal language or wearing any clothing that was reflective of their nation. The goal was to forcibly assimilate Native American children into majority American culture. Yet, it was not until 1924 that American Indians became citizens of the United States.

Ellis Island & Immigration

There were over thirty seven million immigrants who passed through Ellis Island between 1892 and 1954, when it closed. Immigrants came for a variety of reasons, including political and economic stability, religious freedom, and family reunification. During World War I, Ellis Island was used as a site for suspected enemy aliens who were then transferred to other facilities. In the 1920s public sentiment and politicians were beginning to voice concerns over the increased number of immigrants entering the United States. Restrictive laws, similar to The Chinese Exclusion Act and The Alien Contract Labor Law, along with the initiation of a literacy test, helped to deter the aspiring newcomers. The 1924 the National Origins Act limited the number of immigrants each year to two percent of any current ethnic group. The largest number of the immigrant spots were allocated to those coming from Northern and Western Europe, the least from Southern and Eastern Europe. The Act prohibited those entering from Asia altogether. Due to the current labor shortage, there were no restriction for Mexico. (U.S. Department of the Interior).

So why bring up past events that now appear resolved?

History, one's story, may influence decisions about seeking healthcare – trust and relationship being key issues. These histories had an impact on health outcomes.

Recent History . . .

Reflective Exercise: Were you or your parents or grandparents alive when . . .
1. *Dams were built on the Salt & Gila rivers in Arizona in the 1920s?*
2. *Executive Order 9066 was enacted February 19, 1942?*
3. *Port Chicago experienced a munitions explosion on July 17, 1944?*
4. *The Civil Rights Act of 1964 & Voting Rights Act of 1965 were signed?*
5. *Refugees from the Vietnam war immigrated in the 1970s & 1980s?*
6. *Which of these events were experienced by your patients? . . What impact do you think it had?*

It is thought that events of the recent past have the most impact on our lives. Why? The answer may lie in the fact that if we were alive during that time, our response to the events was personalized. In addition, we saw and interpreted each event through our cultural lens. If you were a Native American living in the Southwest, the building of dams impacted your families' ability to farm the land. If you were a Japanese American living on the west coast, loss of business and property due to the enactment of Executive Order 9066 (National Archives) is part of your memory. As an African American, the Civil Rights movement and struggle to obtain equal rights were witnessed in the marches and protests. Each person takes a recent event and internalizes it. Memories may include wariness of government and of those in healthcare institutions. As we reflect on our patient population, we realize that, seen through their eyes, the story may take a different perspective. Let's take a brief look at each.

Construction of dams in the Southwestern portion of the United States had a significant health impact on the Native American nations residing in that area. By 1930, dams had been erected on the Salt and Gila rivers of Arizona. Land once used by the local tribes for farming and fishing was no longer available, and those activities came to an abrupt halt. No longer able to provide for themselves, Native Americans grew to rely on government food subsidies and a sedentary lifestyle.

Japanese Internment followed the bombing of Pearl Harbor on December 7, 1941. On February 19, 1942, President Franklin Roosevelt signed Executive Order 9066, authorizing the Secretary of War to define military areas "from which any or all persons may be excluded as deemed necessary or desirable." The only significant opposition would come from the Quakers (Society of Friends) and the American Civil Liberties Union. Over 122,000 Japanese, many of them citizens of the United States, were forced to live in makeshift housing predominately in the high desert areas away from the Pacific coastline. Manzanar, a site in the Owens Valley, was home to many who had previously lived and owned property and profitable businesses on the west coast. When I toured this site, it became abundantly clear that sanitary and health conditions were questionable. There was little room for privacy. Release from these sites came at the conclusion of World War II. On February 18, 1999, the Justice Department installed a $1.6 billion reparation program for ethnic Japanese interned in American camps during World War II.

The Chicago Port Naval Magazine explosion occurred on July 17, 1944. Of the three hundred and twenty killed, two hundred and two were African American. Following the event two hundred and fifty African Americans refused to return to work, citing unsafe conditions. Fifty leaders were identified, charged with mutiny, and imprisoned. In 1946 they were released without amnesty. Finally in 1992, a pardon was granted to Freddie Meeks, one of the last two survivors. In the San Francisco Chronicle (Franko 2007) a story appeared marking the anniversary of the event. A woman by the name of Diana McDaniel was featured in the article. She stated that she "heard this story as a child." She was advocating that a center be established because "the story cannot be told enough. . . ." Recent history is passed down from one generation to the next. It had been sixty years since that event, but the story continues to be told. In 2009 President Barak Obama designated the site as a National Memorial.

The Civil Rights Act of 1964 and the **Voting Rights Act of 1965** were enacted to ensure the rights of all people of the United States. It had been a hundred years since the passage of the 13th, 14th, and 15th amendments, and yet in some parts of the country, discriminatory practices were still prevalent. Separate schools and separate entrances for blacks and other minorities had been the norm. Separate hospitals were set up in the late 1880s at the request of the American Medical Association and were in existence until the late 1970s. Separate, however, did not equate with equal services.

The Tuskegee study which began in 1941 engendered a great deal of distrust of those conducting health research. Participants of this study, African American men, were not provided treatment for syphilis even though there was a known cure at the time. The hesitancy to seek care today may be part of the reason for health disparities found in the African American population. This study is a prime example that has, for some, led to mistrust of most healthcare professionals.

Manuel Pablo fought with the Americans to protect the Philippines during World War II and participated in the Bataan Death March. At the time he was promised citizenship, a pension and medical benefits, along with resident rights for himself and his children. In a recent article (McAvoy 2007) Mr. Pablo stated that those rights were not realized until 1990 with a revision in the Immigration Act of 1964, which now allows him to bring only one family member to the United States. His other children have been on the wait list for a visa for thirteen years. In her book *The Spirit Catches You and You Fall Down,* Anne Fadimen (1996) cites that some Hmong men who served with the United States military during the Vietnam War, believed that they, too, would receive veteran benefits following their emigration to America. That did not prove to be a reality. As HCP's, we can help to change a negative experience to a positive one by recognizing their contribution to American society and honoring their individual cultures.

Today ~ Being present with the present

History has a way of repeating itself. We, as HCP's, have the opportunity to change the course of events, especially when it comes to the care and treatment of our patient population. Acknowledging the fact that the persons we serve may not trust the health system, we are in a unique position to dialogue about this with them. We must recognize that injustices have occurred, and continue to address issues of prejudice and discrimination when we see them. The journey to cultural competence begins with an awareness that past events may influence present encounters with patients and colleagues as well. Realizing that these events may have occurred three hundred years ago, sixty years ago, or yesterday admonishes us to be vigilant in all our encounters, communications and actions.

Resources

Appel, S.J. (2013). Vietnamese Americans. In J.N. Giger (Eds.) *Transcultural Nursing: Assessment and Intervention.* (6th Ed.) Missouri: Elsevier Mosby

Burns, K., Duncan, D. (2009). The National Parks: America's Best Idea. Public Broadcasting System.

California Newsreel. (2008). Unnatural Causes: Is inequality making us sick?

Center for Disease Control and Prevention. U.S. Public Health Service Syphilis Study at Tuskegee. Retrieved November 24, 2009 from www.cdc.gov/tuskegee.

Cherry, B., Giger, J.N. (2013). African Americans. In J.N. Giger (Ed.) *Transcultural Nursing: Assessment and Intervention.* (6th Ed.) St Louis Missouri: Elsevier Mosby

Conti, K.M. (2006). Diabetes prevention in Indian country: Developing nutrition models to tell the story of food-system change. *Journal of Transcultural Nursing.* (17)3, 234-245.

Fadiman, A. (1996). *The Spirit Catches You and You Fall Down.* New York: Farrar, Straus and Giroux.

Falicov. C.J. (2005). Mexican Families. In M.M. McGoldrick, J. Giordano, Garcia-Preto, N. (Eds.). *Ethnicity and Family Therapy.* (3rd Ed.). New York: Guilford Press.

Farmworkers Organization. The Bracero Program. Retrieved August 2, 2009 from www.farmworkers.org/bracero.

Franko, K. (2007). New bill keeps Port Chicago's story alive. *San Francisco San Francisco Chronicle.* July 30, 2007.

Giger, J.N., Appel, S.J., Davidhizar, R.E., Davis, C. (2008). Church and spirituality in the lives of the African American community. *Journal of Transcultural Nursing.* (19)4, 375-383.

Campinha-Bacote (2013). People of African American ancestry. In L.D. Purnell (Ed.) *Transcultural Health Care.* (4th Ed.). Philadelphia PA: F.A. Davis.

Giordano, J., McGoldrick, M. (2005). European Families: An Overview. In M. McGoldrick, J. Giordano, Garcia-Preto, N. (Eds.). *Ethnicity & Family Therapy.* (3rd Ed.). New York: The Guilford Press.

Hanley, C.E. (2013). Navajos. In J.N. Giger (Ed). *Transcultural Nursing: Assessment and Intervention.* (6th Ed.). Missouri: Elsevier Mosby

Hines, P.M., Boyd-Franklin, N. (2005). African American Families. In M. McGoldrick, J.Giordano, Garcia-Preto, N. (Eds). *Ethnicity and Family Therapy.* (3rd Ed.) New York: The Guilford Press.

Lee, E., Mock, M.R. (2005). Chinese Families. In M.M. McGoldrick, J. Giordano, Garcia-Preto, N. (Eds.). *Ethnicity and Family Therapy.* (3rd Ed.), New York: Guilford Press.

Leung, P.K., Boehnlein, J. (2005). Vietnamese Families. In M. McGoldrick, J.Giordano, Garcia-Preto, N. (Eds) *Ethnicity and Family Therapy.* (3rd Ed.), New York: The Guilford Press

Lincoln, B. (2010). *Reflections from Common Ground: Cultural Awareness in Healthcare.* Wisconsin: PesiHealthcare

Mann, C. (2005). *1491: New Revelations about Americans before Columbus.* NewYork: Random House.

Malthus, T. (1798). Essay on Principles of Population. Retrieved on July 1, 2009 from www.espy.org/books/malthus/population.

McGill, D.W., Pearce, J.K. (2005). American Families with English Ancestors from the Colonial Era: Anglo Americans. In M.MGoldrick, J. Giordano, N. Garcia-Preto (Eds.) *Ethnicity & Family Therapy.* (3rd Ed.). New York: The Guilford Press.

McGoldrick, M., Giordano, J., Garcia-Preto, N. (2005). *Ethnicity & Family Therapy.* (3rd Ed.). New York: The Guilford Press.

McAvoy, A. (2007). Aging Filipino WWII Veterans forced to live apart from families. *San Francisco Chronicle.* March 18, 2007.

National Park Service. Ellis Island. Retrieved October 3, 2009 from www.nps.gov. National Archives.

U.S. Constitution. Retrieved March 20, 2010 from www.archieves.com

National Archives. Executive Order 9066. Retrieved August 2, 2009 from www.archives.com

Mattson, S (2013). People of Vietnamese heritage. In L.D. Purnell (Ed.) *Transcultural Health Care.* (4th Ed.). Philadelphia PA: F.A. Davis.

Owen, D.C., Gonzalez, E.W., Esperat, C.R. (2013). Mexican Americans. In J.N. Giger (Ed) *Transcultural Nursing: Assessments and Interventions.* (6th Ed.) New York: Elsevier Mosby

Spector, R. (2012). *Cultural Diversity in Health and Illness.* (8th Ed.) New Jersey: Pearson, Prentice Hall.

Staisak, D. (1991). Culture care theory with Mexican Americans in an urban context. In M.M. Leininger (Ed.). *Culture care diversity & universality: A theory in nursing.* New York: National League for Nursing Press.

Still, O., Hodgins, D. (2003). Navajo Indians. In L.D. Purnell, B.J. Paulanks (Eds.) *Transcultural health care: A culturally competent approach.*(2nd Ed.). Philadelphia, PA: F.A. Davis

Penner, L.A., Dovidio, J.F., Edmondson, D., Dailey, R.K., Markova, T., Albrecht, T.L., Gaertner, S.L. (2009). The experience of discrimination and Black-White health disparities in medical care. *Journal of Black Psychology.* (35)2. Pp: 181-203.

United States Department of State. Public Diplomacy & Public Affairs. Retrieved on November 24, 2009 from www.state.gov.

United States Department of the Interior. Bureau of Indian Affairs. Retrieved Retrieved November 24, 2009 from www.cr.nps.gov.

United States Department of the Interior. Ellis Island: History and Culture. Retrieved October 20, 2009 from www.nps.gov/ellis/historyculture.

Wang, Y. (2008). People of Chinese Heritage. In L.D. Purnell, B.J. Paulanka (Eds). *Transcultural Health Care: A Culturally Competent Approach.* (3rd Ed.), Philadelphia: F.A. Davis.

Warne, D. (2006). Research and educational approaches to reducing health disparities among American Indians and Alaskan natives. *Journal of Transcultural Nursing.* (17)3, 266-271.

Xu, Y, Chang, K. (2013). Chinese Americans. In J.N. Giger (Ed). *Transcultural Nursing: Assessments andInterventions.* (6th Ed.), New York: Elsevier Mosby

Zoucha, R., Zamarripa, C. (2013). People of Mexican Heritage. In L.D. Purnell (Ed). *Transcultural Health Care: A Culturally Competent Approach.* (4th Ed.).Philadelphia: F.A. Davis.

Growing More Diverse ...Trends Over Time | 3

"... demographics are only as good as the people who fill out the forms"

~ A seminar participant

This was the response I received during a recent seminar. A participant, sitting at the back of the room and acting as though he wished he was somewhere else, startled me with is response. But, he was right! The census data is only as reliable as the people who fill out the forms. Much has been written about the hesitancy of some to provide the information because of illiteracy, distrust, or apathy toward the process. What the census does reflect is trends over time.

The census was written into the United States Constitution of 1789 and stated:

Article I, Section 2
of the Constitution of the United States

"Representation and direct Taxes shall be apportioned among the several States which may be included within this Union, according to their respective Numbers ... , The actual Enumeration shall be made within three Years after the first Meeting of the Congress of the United States, and within every subsequent Term of ten Years, in such Manner as they shall by Law direct."

It came about because the Revolutionary War created a debt. No longer receiving support from England, the Congress looked to the new states to share the debt and to provide revenue. In addition, it gave an accurate picture of the current population, which determined representation in Congress. The initial census included "white" males and excluded Indians who were not taxed. Slaves were counted as 3/5 of a person. Each succeeding census in the 1800s saw a 25% to 30% growth in population. The 3/5 slave designation was repealed in 1865 with the passage of the 14th Amendment. In 1913, the 16th Amendment authorized direct taxation of the individual which ended the census' role in determining state taxation.

The current census includes White and Black (African American, Negro); those identifying as American Indian or Alaskan Native can list their tribe affiliation; Spanish/ Hispanic/Latino can list Mexican, Mexican American, Chicano, Puerto Rican, Cuban or write in another group. Those of Asian or Southeast Asian heritage are also given an opportunity to write in another race. So yes, we definitely see trends over time, and that enables us to reflect on the changes within out community and country.

U.S. Census Bureau Population 2013

Black ~ African American	12.2%
American Indian/Alaskan Native	0.7%
Asian	4.8%
Native Hawaiian/ Pacific Islander	0.2%
Hispanic ~ Latino	16.6%
White ~ Non Hispanic	63.3%

Who fits in what category . . . interesting!

According to the U.S. Census Bureau (2010) the "concept of race reflects self-identification by people according to the race or races with which they most closely identify. These categories are sociopolitical constructs and should not be interpreted as being scientific or anthropological in nature. Furthermore, the race categories include both racial and national-origin groups."

The following race classification used by the U.S. Census Bureau is consistent with the "Revisions to the Standards for the Classification of Federal Data on Race and Ethnicity" issued in 1997 by the Office of Management and Budget. Each group listed below includes both race and national-origin as the defining factors.

White: a person having origins in any of the original peoples of Europe, the Middle East or North Africa. It includes people who indicate their race as "White" or other such as Irish, German, Lebanese, Arab, and Polish.

Black or African American: a person having origins in any of the Black racial groups of Africa. It includes those who indicate their race as "Black, African American, or Negro" or provide written entries such as Nigerian, Afro American, Kenyan, and Haitian.

American Indian and Alaskan Native: a person having origins in any of the original peoples of North and South America (including Central America) and who maintain tribal affiliation or community attachment.

Asian: a person having origins in any of the original peoples of the Far East, Southeast Asia, or the Indian subcontinent including for example, Cambodia, China, India, Japan, Korea, Malaysia, Pakistan, the Philippine Islands, Thailand and Vietnam. It includes Asian Indian, Chinese, Filipino, Korean, Japanese, Vietnamese, and Other Asian.

Native Hawaiian and Other Pacific Islander: a person having origins in any of the original peoples of Hawaii, Guam, Samoa, or other Pacific Islands. It includes people who indicate their race as Native Hawaiian, Guamanian or Chamorro, Samoan, and Other Pacific Islander.

> *Reflective Exercise: Who lives here... works here...?*
> 1. *What is the demographic make up of your community?*
> 2. *Is this a change from ten or twenty years ago?*
> 3. *Do you have an immigrant or refugee population?*
> 4. *Are healthcare professionals representative of your patient population?*

Immigrants and health

The article, *America's Diversity at the Beginning of the 21st Century: Reflections from Census 2000*, written by Audrey Singer (2002) of the Brooking Institution, explores the similarities and differences between the immigrants arriving at the beginning of the 20th century and those coming at the end. In the early 1900s Southern and Eastern Europeans constituted the majority of immigrants, 14.5 million, admitted to the United States. The end of the century found that the majority of groups came from Asia, Latin American, the Caribbean, and Africa. Singer states that "both periods – the beginning and the end of the century – have been characterized by a broad restructuring of the nation's economy, from agricultural to industry in the early period and in the later period from manufacturing to services and information technology."

More than a million immigrants come to this country annually, many seeking a better life for themselves and their families. According to the 2013 American Community Survey there are over forty-two million foreign born persons living in the United States - 48% naturalized citizens and 53% are not citizens. The majority, or 52%, come from the Latin Americas, 30% from Asia, 12% from Europe and 5% from African. Generally there are more men than women. Their ages ranges from 18 and 64. In addition, there are over 12 million undocumented immigrants in the United States. While this constitutes less than 0.4% of the total population it seems to generate the majority of attention with regard to healthcare, education and employment.

Let's look at the health of one immigrant group. The California Newsreel documentary *Unnatural Causes . . . Is Inequality Making Us Sick* (2008) cites that Latino immigrants have the *best health* in the country – better health than the wealthiest. The authors hypothesized two reasons for this finding: (1) only the healthiest make it across the border; and (2) the role of strong cohesive ties with family and strong social networks that form a protective barrier. Unfortunately, though, within one generation those same health advantages decline. Acculturation, adapting to the American way of life, may lead to intergenerational stress and a loss of connection with family. The health protective benefits begin to wane and health issues such as obesity, diabetes and heart disease rise.

> *Reflective exercise: Immigrants in your community*
> 1. *Who are the immigrants in your community? Are you familiar with their cultural beliefs and health care practices?*
> 2. *What challenges you the most when caring for this population?*
> 3. *What resources are available...for you...for your patients?*
> 4. *Has your organization provided you with continuing education programs to care for diverse populations?*

HCP Demographics . . . are they changing?

As the demographic landscape continues to change, the challenge facing HCPs is providing culturally sensitive and competent care. The current HCP population, however, is predominately white. The following data highlights the numbers: Health Resources and Services Administration (HRSA 2010) shows the registered nurse population; the Office of Minority Health (2004), the physician population; and the Center for Workforce Studies & National Association of Social Workers (2004), the social worker demographics. The numbers are rounded up.

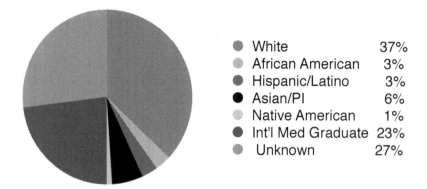

Figure 3-1 Registered Nurse Demographics

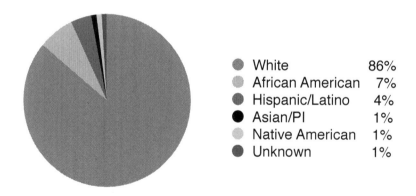

Figure 3-2: Physician Demographics

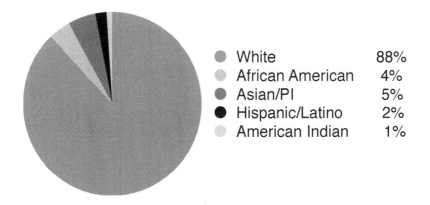

Figure 3-3: Social Workers Demographics

Finding the future HCP...

According to the National League of Nursing (2008), 24% of all nursing graduates nationally are minorities: Black 10.3%, Hispanic 7%, Asian/PI 4.5%, American Indian 1%, and other 3.7%. Enrollment in medical schools, similar to that of registered nurses, shows minimal increase for all minority groups with the exception of Hispanics which is declining. Unfortunately, this leads to an under representation of bilingual and bicultural HCPs in hospitals, clinics and home health programs.

Legislation entitled Closing the Health Care Gap, passed by Congress in 2004, addressed the need for more diversity in the healthcare field by funding outreach programs to attract minority students. Yet, why does there continue to be a disparity in the HCP demographics? For those minority students in high school considering a career in healthcare, the educational level and income of their parents may be a factor. Navigating the college application process and facing limited funding can adversely affect their ability to follow their dream. Language proficiency for students who have been here less than five years, may seem like an insurmountable obstacle.

In the article *Racial/Ethnic Disparities in Nursing* (2001), Coffman, Rosenoff, and Grumback hypothesize that one reason for low enrollment of minority groups in college may be due to low rates of high school graduation. According to the Brooking Institution Civil Rights Report of 2004, there is a fifty percent dropout rate for African Americans, Latinos, and American Indians. Those who do pursue higher education may be less likely than Whites to obtain a degree in nursing. If this is the current reality, then what can we do to change that trend? It may be as simple as serving as a role model to the young people we meet or helping present at health fairs at their schools. Share your passion for what you do and let students know they can make a difference in the lives of others. Getting young people interested and excited earlier, rather than later, may be the key to increasing the diversity of HCP's in the future. When we inspire and motivate, young people listen and are encouraged to further their education.

Other barriers for future HCPs . . . perhaps

Cultural beliefs and value may influence one's decision to enter the healthcare field. Those in the American Indian culture may view nursing as undesirable because it involves being around sick people. Olivia Still and David Hodgins (2003) share that most of the nurses in the Indian Health Service are not American Indian. They went on to note that "It is frequently said that if an American Indian became a physician, he must not be 'traditional' .". . . therefore many Navajo are suspicious of American Indian physicians."[2]

Those who value harmony and are more collectivistic than individualistic, such as the Native Hawaiian, may view the classroom and clinical areas as competitive, aggressive, and unwelcoming. At a recent Transcultural Nursing Society conference, a registered nurse, who was also native Hawaiian, shared the story of her university experience. In the classroom, she said "None of the Hawaiians would ever speak, but when they attended separate classes just for their group they never stopped talking and sharing." She felt intimidated by the individual competition. and was more comfortable working in a group. This style is consistent with her cultural values and educational practices. That experience was ten years ago, but she shared it with me as if it happened yesterday.

Another limitation may be related to religious values and beliefs that prevent providing care to a person of the opposite sex (Muslim and Orthodox Jew), or working certain days of the week such as the sabbath (Seventh Day Adventist, Muslim, Orthodox Jew). These limitations may restrict the ability of the student to become a full participant in the educational process.

Creating a welcoming environment

Acknowledging the need and the opportunity for a more diverse healthcare staff, we need to recognize the ambiance of the academic arena which sets the stage for student success. Clinical experiences challenge the students' ability to transition academic knowledge to clinical practice. Do you remember your first day as a student or as a new graduate? Even though we were apprehensive, our expectations were high. The encouragement we received from the veteran staff helped to make it a success. The most important thing we can do is to provide a supportive and welcoming environment.

Moving on . . .

As a country we are becoming more diverse. We are a destination for many immigrants and refugees. This will continue. HCPs, at this time, do not reflect the current population. As HCPs, we grapple with the unknown, the uncertainty, and the challenges of working and caring for people from diverse ethnic, cultural, and religious backgrounds. My colleagues say "It's about the patient . . . the patient comes first." We need to do what is necessary to provide care and restore health and well-being. Are we ready?

Resources

Association of American Medical Colleges. (2006). American Needs a More Diverse Physician Workforce. AAMC: Washington D.C.

Coffman, J.M., Rosenoff, E., Grumbach. K. (2001). Racial/Ethnic Disparities in Nursing. Health Affairs. May/June 263-264.Ed.). Missouri: Elsevier Mosby

California Newsreel. (2008). Unnatural causes . . . Is inequality making us sick. www.unnaturalcauses.org.

Hendricks, T. (2009). Kids Boost Diversity as State Ages. San Francisco Chronicle.

Lincoln, B. (2010). *Reflections from Common Ground: Cultural Awareness in Healthcare.* Wisconsin: PesiHealthcare

Lipson, J., Dibble, S., Minarik, P.A. (2001). *Culture & Nursing Care: A Pocket Guide.* (8th Ed.) UCSF Press: San Francisco, CA

National League of Nursing. (2008). Number of nursing school graduates. Retrieved November 23, 2013 from www.nln.org.

NASW Center for Workforce Studies. (2006). Licensed Social Workers in the United States, 2004.

Olvera, M.L. (2005). Fact Sheet: Census Schedules and Ethnic Classification IL: Cultural Marketing Communication and Urban Reach Public Relations.www.culturalmarketingcommunications.com.

Purnell, L.D. (2013). *Transcultural health care: A culturally competent approach.* (4th Ed.). Philadelphia, PA: F.A. Davis Company.

Ryan, C. (2012). Language Use in the United States: 2011. American Community Survey Reports. U.S. Department of Commerce. Economics and Statistic Administration

Singer, A. (2002). America's Diversity at the Beginning of the 21st Century: Reflections from Census 2000. Brooking Institute: Washington D.C. 1-15.

Still, O., Hodgins, D. (2004). Navajo Indians. In L.D. Purnell, B.J. Paulanka (Eds). *Transcultural Health Care: A Culturally Competent Approach.* (3rd Ed). Philadelphia:F.A. Davis.

Spector, R. (2012). *Cultural diversity in health and illness.* (8th Ed.). New Jersey: Pearson/Prentice Hall.

U.S. Department of Health and Human Services. (2005). Minorities in Medicine: An Ethnic and Cultural Challenge for Physician Training. Council on Graduate Medical Education 17th Report. 1-62

U.S. Department of Health Resources and Services Administration. (2010). The Register Nurse Population: National Sample Survey of Registered Nurses. Retrieved June 17, 2016 from http: www.hrsa.gov/healthworkforce/rnsurvey

It's time to have the Conversation . . .

4

> "But race is an issue that I believe this nation cannot afford to ignore right now . . ."
>
> Barak Obama - Mach 3, 2008

And that comment is even more relevant today. It is time to have the conversation! Most find racism, prejudice, and discrimination difficult topics at best and would rather avoid them or pretend that they don't exist: but they do exist. Each one may influence a person's access to care, treatment, and health outcomes. The authors of the documentary entitled *Unnatural Causes: Is Inequality Making Us Sick?* aired by PBS in 2009 believed that constant exposure to racism and discrimination increases stress and has a negative impact on one's health. The body's physiological response to stress is to release large amounts of cortisol from the adrenal glands. While this is helpful in a "fight or flight' situation," continuous release results in an elevation of blood pressure and blood sugar while lowering the immune system. So, yes, we need to talk about this subject, to identify biases and to eliminate prejudice, discrimination, and racism for many reasons including our own health.

Race ... Why did it begin ..?

Let's look at the word race from an historical perspective. The term was constructed in the mid to late 1800s during a time when all things were being categorized, thus systematically explaining the surroundings. Race is a social construct, not necessarily based on ethnicity, but more significantly on the color of one's skin (2006 American Anthropological Association). Scientists used the taxonomic system to classify humans during this period of time, positing that there were biological differences in capabilities and intellect. It provided the legitimacy for laws that promoted social inequalities, thus disenfranchising groups of people such as African Americans, American Indians, immigrants and others.

Racism and other uncomfortable subjects

Racism, unfortunately alive and well, is demonstrated through acts of prejudice and discrimination. It may be subtle. It may be overt. Think about a time when you experienced some form of racism. How did you feel? What did you do? How did it change your perspective of the individual or organization involved? Dr. Adewale Troutman, Public Health and Wellness Director in Louisville Kentucky, shares his story in the PBS series *Unnatural Causes . . .Is Inequality Making Us Sick*. He serves a county populated by Kentucky's poor and disenfranchised. Yet, as an African American, he has experienced racism where he lives and works. "There are times when I get on the elevator and the elderly white women clutches her purse . . . or every time I walk down the aisles of a certain store someone follows me to make sure I am not stealing anything. What they don't know about me is that I live in an affluent part of the city and hold two degrees," he said in the documentary previously cited. Many people face this every day and as HCPs our antennas must be attuned to incidents that occur in our workplace.

Let's review the following definitions and reflect on their impact on ourselves, our patients, and our colleagues.

- Race ~ a sociopolitical construct; refers to the genetic, biological differences such as skin color, or other outward physical appearances
- Racism ~ a belief that all members of each race possess certain characteristics or abilities specific to that race; especially to distinguish it as inferior or superior to another race or races
- Ethnicity ~ a group that shares a common history, culture, values and beliefs, linguistic or religious beliefs along with other characteristics that form a shared identity
- Prejudice ~ a set of rigid and unfavorable attitudes toward a particular individual or group that is formed without consideration of facts
- Discrimination ~ a set of attitudes that often leads to the differential treatment of individuals or groups based on categories such as race, ethnicity, gender, sexual orientation, social class, religious affiliation, immigrant status.
- Cultural bias ~ believing that one's personal beliefs and values are superior
- Cultural imposition ~ imposing one's cultural beliefs and values on another in an intrusive manner
- Ethnocentrism ~ the belief, assumption or perception that oneself or group is superior to another; an inherent superiority

Forming opinions . . . it begins early in life

We learn biases at a early age. Prior to one's ability to differentiate between races of people, observation and socialization with our family of origin lay the groundwork for establishing biases. Before the age of five a child learns attitudes and beliefs about the differences between people and the things in their environment. Recently, a five year old child whose mother is white and father is black, shared an 'aha' moment when he said to his mother, "I know who I am . . . it's kinda like ice cream. I am chocolate, because I am dark; you are vanilla because you are white; and Sammy (his younger brother) is," and here he paused, "Sammy is marble fudge, because he is more white than black." He had selected something that he loved, ice cream, and used it to provide positive attributes to his mother and brother. By the age of ten this same child will likely form attitudes and beliefs – positive and negative about ethnic groups. This is what his world tells him about the "other" and he begins to believe it to be true. It is not until adulthood, however, that one has the opportunity to change previous biases, behaviors, and stereotypical opinions about others.

Bias . . . Naming it . . . Saying it . . . Dissolving it

Bias, negative or positive; conscious or unconscious, is a belief about a particular subject or people. This then translates into stereotyping – a firmly held belief that influences how one interacts with another.

> *Reflective exercise: List your first positive & negative thoughts . .*
> 1. *African American - college - male - dreadlocks*
> 2. *Asian - math - herbs - driving*
> 3. *White - pregnant - poverty - alone*
> 4. *American Indian - overweight - casino - pride*
> 5. *Woman - executive - African American - new*
> 6. *Elderly - new hire - thrifty - organized*

What was the first thought that came into your head after reading each one? Did some of your responses surprise you? If this had been done in a group setting, different perspectives would have been presented. Those responses can help us to widen our views and open us to a new way of thinking, thus hopefully eliminating previously held biases and stereotypes.

Stereotyping as defined by Webster's 1950 Merriam Dictionary refers to the use of a mold to make a plate . . lacking originality or individuality . . to repeat without variation; to hackney. The 2009 version defines stereotyping as "oversimplification of the typical characteristics of a person or thing." The difference of sixty years takes the term to a new level. Research in social psychology indicates that stereotyping is a *universal cognitive function* (IOM 2002). It is not unique to one group of people, one religious sect, or one socioeconomic group. It is universal and worldwide. On a recent trip to Costa Rica for a Spanish immersion program, mi madre (in Costa Rica) told me about the *Nicas* and the *Ticas*. Still not well versed in Spanish, I asked for clarification. She informed me, en Español, that the *Ticas* were Costa Ricans and the *Nicas* were Nicaraguans. The *Nicas* were coming across the border to use Costa Rica's health facilities, schools, and welfare system. Being naïve I asked "How can you tell the difference?" She adamantly shared "They all (she place great emphasis on the word all) look and talk the same." A recent documentary on immigrants entering Botswana from Zimbabwe depicted a similar view that these immigrants were taking jobs and using resources. How could they tell the difference between the those from Botswana and those from Zimbabwe? The response from one woman: "They smell different." In her worldview it was fact. What we see and what we know may be very different. .

Why do we do this? Initially, it may provide confidence in our ability to control the situation or possibly to be used to respond when facts are not readily available. Unfortunately it may create and promote validation of opinions which are prejudiced. The Institute of Medicine (IOM) report *Unequal Treatment* (2002) states that research in cognitive psychology reveal that stereotypes:

- Are automatically activated ~ generated without conscious effort
- Are held by people who truly believe they do not judge others
- Affect how we process and recall information about others
- Guide our expectations and perceptions and shape our personal interaction

The Proverbial "Iceberg"

The proverbial "iceberg" is a frequently used image that helps us to understand that much of what we do not know about patients and colleagues is beneath the water line, yet to be discovered. Initial encounters may evoke positive and negative opinions. Our patients may have an iceberg perspective of us as well. Based on previous encounters with other health professionals, the patient may draw on her memory to form an opinion. It is vital that we as HCP's understand that our patients present to us with their biases as well.

The more knowledge HCPs have about cultural values, beliefs, healthcare practices of various ethnic groups, the more likely they are to have established respectful and trusting relationships with patients and colleagues.

- Knowledge replaces stereotyping
- Positive and respectful encounters replace stereotyping
- Welcoming environments replace stereotyping

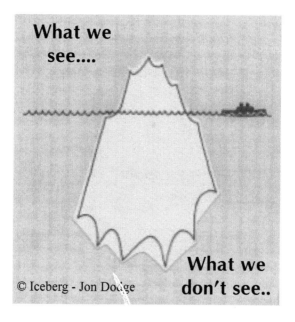

Figure 4-Iceberg©

Overcoming bias in the every day

Biases can lead to making decisions that negatively affect future encounters. So what are the steps one should take to elevate consciousness, address the bias, and then eliminate it? *Reducing Unconscious Bias* (2009), an article by Sondra Thiederman, Ph.D. (copyright 2009 Sondra Thiederman/Cross-Cultural Communications; www.thiederman.com used with permission) offers the following suggestions:

- **Step 1: Become aware of your bias**
  - Identify that first thought that comes to mind when encountering someone different than yourself
  - What assumptions are you making?

- **Step 2: Examine your thoughts**
  - Look at your reaction and think ~ "would I feel the same way about the meaning of this incident if that person were from a different group?"
  - Is this related to a previous experience with the group involved?
  - If your assumption is incorrect?

- **Step 3: Dissect your bias to reveal its weak foundation**
  - Was the original source of my bias reliable?
  - Was it a self-fulfilling prophecy or the filter of expectation?

- **Step 4: Fake it until you make it**
  - Make a list of the things your bias about how people communicate is causing you to do; and consequence of these behaviors
  - Substitute behavior and visualize positive consequences
  - The more positive one views another, the better response from that individual and the more positive the experience for all concerned.

Thiederman suggests *Bias Spotter Partnerships* which is based on the following four principles: (1) awareness of our biases is the best first step toward resolution, (2) human beings resist identifying our own biases because we feel that having a bias means we are bad people, (3) the stress and rush of the workplace deprives us of the luxury of spotting the tiny clues to bias that our behavior and thoughts reveal, and (4) team members can serve as trusted aids in bringing about awareness of our biases. This approach can be used in the workplace and thus translates into a collaborative effort in which all members of the team/staff identify biases in the spirit of mutual support without being accusatory. Confidentiality is important as well. For the next couple of weeks, notice the first thought that comes into your mind when encountering someone different than yourself or that patient with a long history of negative encounters with HCPs. Use the four steps outlined to identify, examine, dissect and substitute previous behavior and thoughts. You will see new and positive outcomes. Attitude follows behavior.

Ethnocentrism & Cultural Acceptance

Juxtaposing these two terms may seem an oxymoron, but in reality one may actually lead to another. Ethnocentrism, according to W.G. Summer in the early part of the 20th century, was defined as "the view of things in which one's own group is the center of everything and all others are scaled and rated from it."[3] It is interesting to note that he suggests that persons hold onto these beliefs, values, and folkways in order to protect themselves from foreigners. It was a survival strategy to maintain one's identity.

Cultural values and practices learned as a child through observation, communication, and socialization can lead to ethnocentric beliefs. Becoming aware that one has beliefs of superiority over another individual or group, provides the first step in the journey to ethnorelativism, a belief that another's cultural beliefs, values, and ways of living in the world are on a equal par with one's own. This transition does not happen in a day, a week, or a year. It does not happen because of one incident, one encounter, or one "aha" moment. Opportunities to learn about others garners cultural knowledge and moves us from the unconscious ethnocentric thoughts to a conscious decision to make changes that will lead to culturally sensitive and competent healthcare.

Our patients also may hold ethnocentric beliefs about us. Expectations may lead to misunderstandings, tension, and uncertainty. It is during these moments that we realize that this is an opportunity to dispel previously held biases and eliminate stereotyping of each other. When we persevere in difficult times, we learn something new about our patients and ourselves.

Now to assessment . . .

Where are you on the river of prejudice and discrimination. This activity allows recognition that a response may vary according to the situation. Visualize yourself in a canoe on a river. Yes, you have a life jacket on ~ a great metaphor for dealing in uncertainty. There are five potential answers, beginning with Level 1, promoting racism and discrimination, to Level 5 in which you are a constant voice speaking out against injustice. Where are you?

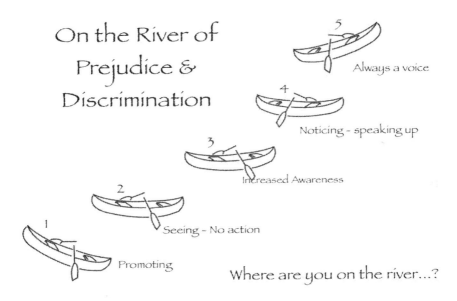

Figure 4-2: On the River

Reflective exercise: Where are you on the river . . . ?					
1. *In the clinical setting:*	*1*	*2*	*3*	*4*	*5*
2. *In the staff meeting:*	*1*	*2*	*3*	*4*	*5*
3. *At the supermarket:*	*1*	*2*	*3*	*4*	*5*
4. *At a family gathering:*	*1*	*2*	*3*	*4*	*5*

Where to from here . . .

The process is ongoing. Take the opportunity to attend cultural awareness education seminars that address issues of prejudice, discrimination and racism in addition to cultural beliefs, values, and practices of various groups. Reviewing policies and procedures, orientation programs, staff evaluations, annual goals and objectives, and the mission statement of the organization can and should be part of this process. It's time to talk about all things uncomfortable!

Resources

American Anthropological Association. (2006). The Story of Race. Retrieved October 5, 2009 from http://w.w.w..understandingrace.com.

American College of Obstetricians and Gynecologist. (2011). Committee Opinion:Cultural Sensitivity and awareness in the delivery of health care. 117:1258-61.

Andrews, M.M., Boyle, J.S. (2016). *Transcultural concepts in nursing care.* (7th Ed.). New York: Wolters Kluwer.

Campinha-Bacote, J. (2003). *The process of cultural competence in the delivery of healthcare services: A culturally competent model of care.* Cincinnati, OH: Transcultural C.A.R.E. Associates

Beckles, G. (2008). The intellectual origins of race. Retrieved November 5, 2008 from www.suite101.com.

Capell, J., Dean, E., Veenstra, G. (2008). The relationship between cultural competence and ethnocentrism of health care professionals. *Journal of Transcultural Nursing.* (19)2; 121-125.

Galanti, G. (2015). *Caring for Patients from Different Cultures.* Pennsylvania: University of Pennsylvania Press.

Giger, J.N. (2013). *Transcultural nursing: Assessment and intervention.* (6th Ed.). Missouri: Elsevier Mosby.

Giger, J., Davidhizar, R., Purnell, L., Harden, J., Phillips, J., Stickland. (2007). American Academy of Nursing Expert Panel Report: Developing cultural competence to eliminate health disparities in ethnic minorities and other vulnerable populations. *Journal of Transcultural Nursing.* (18) 2, 95-102.

Hassouneh-Phillips, D, Beckett, P. (2003). An education in Racism. *Journal of Nursing Education.* (42)6; 258-266.

Leininger, M.M. (1991). *Culture care diversity and universality: A theory of nursing.* New York:National League for Nursing Press.

Leininger, M.M., McFarland, M.R. (2002). *Transcultural nursing: Concepts, theories, research and practice.* (3rd Ed.). New York: McGraw-Hill.

Lincoln, B. (2010). *Reflections from Common Ground: Cultural Awareness in Healthcare.* Wisconsin: PesiHealthcare

Lipson, J. G., Dibble, S.L., Minarik, P.A. (2001). *Culture & Nursing Care: A pocket guide.* San Francisco: UCSF Nursing Press

Mansour, M. (1994). Cultural circles: Application of Family Systems Theory in staff development. *Journal of Nursing Staff Development.* (10)1; 22-26.

McGoldrick, M., Giordano, J., Garcia-Preto, N. (2005). *Ethnicity and family therapy.* (3rd Ed.) New York: Guilford Press.

Obama, B. (2008). A More Perfect Union. Retrieved on September 14, 2009 from www.huffingtonpost.com.

Purnell, L.D. (2013). *Transcultural health care: A culturally competent approach.* (4th Ed.). Philadelphia, PA: F.A. Davis Company

Smedley, B., Stith, A., Nelson, A. (2002). Unequal treatment: Confronting racial and ethnic disparities in health care. Institute of Medicine. Washington D.C.: The National Academies Press

Spence, D. (2001). Prejudice, paradox, and possibility: Nursing people from cultures other than one's own. *Journal of Transcultural Nursing.* (12) 2, 100-106.

Spector, R. (2012). *Cultural diversity in health and illness.* (8th Ed.), New Jersey: Pearson/Prentice Hall.

Sutherland, L. (2002). Ethnocentrism in a pluralistic society: a concept analysis. *Journal of Transcultural Nursing.* (13)4; 274-281.

Thiedeman, S. (2009). Reducing Unconscious Bias. Retrieved October 2009 from the www.thiedeman.com

Thiedeman, S. (2009). Aren't you overreacting just a bit? . Retrieved August 2009 from the www.thiedeman.com

Thieiasedeman, S. (2009). Leading bias free. Retrieved October 2008. from the www.thiedeman.

Access to Care... What Gets in the Way? | 5

Barriers, while obvious to those outside of the healthcare system, may be less apparent to those of us who work in the clinical setting. We understand the jargon, the culture, and the ways things are done. It seems routine to us. Take a moment and reflect back to your first day on the job. Did you feel out of your element? Did everybody else seem to know what they were doing except you? I remember feeling very inept, asking too many questions (I thought) and wishing it were six months later when all of this would be familiar.

Now, let's think about our patients. For some or most of them, the healthcare world seems daunting as they attempt to maneuver through the system. In this chapter, barriers to healthcare are identified. Join us on this journey as seen through the eyes of our patients. But first, a bit of history.

Healthcare reform then and now

Healthcare reform has been in process for over a hundred years. Each time the issues have been similar – a large number of uninsured people and growing health concerns. Outcomes were the same – healthcare legislation fails to pass. To help understand today's debate about healthcare reform, it is important that we visit the past. In reality it has been at the forefront of many a political discussions from the Healthcare Initiative of President Theodore Roosevelt to the proposal by President Barak Obama.

While the Socialist Party had endorsed a compulsory healthcare program in 1904, it was not until 1912 that the Progressive Party candidate Teddy Roosevelt advocated for national health insurance in his party's platform. "We pledge ourselves to work unceasingly in State and Nation for . . . the protection of home life against the hazards of sickness, irregular employment and old age through the adoption of a system of social insurance adapted to American use" (www.socialsecurity.gov/history). Unfortunately, he lost the election.

In the article, *Health Care Reform and Social Movements in the United States* (2002), Beatrix Hoffman, Ph.D. writes that many of the successful social movements in the 20th century relied on grassroots' participation – people advocating for reform. Healthcare reform movements, however, were headed by academics, economists, and organizations; thus, they were minimally successful.

In 1915, the American Association for Labor Legislation submitted a proposal advocating for health insurance that would protect ill workers against loss of wages and medical costs. This proposal, modeled after programs in Germany and England, received support from the public, but was defeated in Congress. In the 1920s, a group called the Committee on Costs of Medical Care, supported by academics, economists, and physicians, put their confidence in research rather than people. This was defeated.

In 1945, the Wagner-Murray-Dingell Bill was proposed as a national medical insurance program that was to be financed by the social security payroll taxes. While it was supported by the then president Harry S. Truman, it was defeated as well. It was in July of 1965, during President Lyndon Johnson's term, that Medicare, having been worked on for over a decade, was signed into law. Building on that, Richard Nixon in his address to the Congress in 1971, proposed a National Health Strategy that would address the shortcomings in the healthcare system, including access to care, cost, and availability of healthcare professionals. In 1993, President Bill Clinton initiated discussion on healthcare reform as well. While initially applauded, it was later criticized by the congressional members and never got beyond the discussion phase.

That all changed on March 21, 2010, when the House of Representatives passed the Health Care Reform Bill (HR 3590 Patient Protection and Affordable Care Act) that had been submitted to them by the Senate. It was signed into law by President Barack Obama on Tuesday, March 23, 2010. House amendments, which required Senate approval, were passed on March 25, 2010. What started over a hundred years ago was now law.

Yet, there were those who felt that Congress did not have the constitutional authority to require persons to purchase health insurance which was one of the provisions in the law. They took their case to the Supreme Court. On June 28, 2012, in a five to four vote, the court ruled that the health insurance mandate was constitutional. The majority opinion written by Chief Justice John Roberts, stated that the requirement that every American buy health insurance or pay a penalty, was authorized by Congress' power to levy taxes. This law went into effect January 1, 2014. As HCPs, we readily acknowledge that we are part of the solution as well. We have expertise and experience to ensure that patients receive the best healthcare available. Reflect on some of the ways we can open doors and provide care and resources for our patients.

> *Reflective exercise: Thinking outside the box*
> 1. *In what ways can we increase access to care?*
> 2. *Are our hours of operation meeting the needs of our patient population?*
> 3. *Have our interpreters received medical and cultural training?*
> 4. *Do we involve the community in our decision-making process?*
> 5. *Does our educational material meet the learning needs of our patients?*

In addition to insurance, there are other compelling issues that affect access to care including language, education, literacy, acculturation, and availability of bilingual and bicultural healthcare professionals. Recognition of the need and a desire for change are the first steps in the process. In the next section we review each issue and identify ways to eliminate these barriers.

Socioeconomic

Facts are important and set the stage for understanding the magnitude of living in this world in which money and/or income dictates one's ability to meet even the basic needs. Socioeconomics has always played a role in healthcare, as we noted in the healthcare reform section. According to the U.S. Census Report (2013) the median income is now $51,017. The range of incomes varies from a low of $33,321 for African Americans to a high of $68,636 for Asians. Regionally, the West has the highest median household income of $52,376, followed by the Northeast and Midwest, with the South having the lowest income at $46,889. Women make 79 cents on every dollar a man makes. There continues to be economic discrepancies between gender, race, and region which ultimately impacts one's ability to pay for healthcare.

There are over 46 million people living in poverty in the United States. While that may be only 15% of the total population, it still remains that 46 million people wake up to that fact each day. According to the U.S. Census Bureau Report of 2012, the change from the previous census was "not statistically significant." Those who live with poverty would probably put more emphasis on the word "significant." While other aspects of their life may be within their power to control, finances are not. Let's look more closely at those who live at or below the poverty level.

Poverty in the United States[4]

American Indian/Alaskan Native	26%
African American	27.2%
Hispanic	23/5%
Asian	10.5%
White	9.6%

Currently for a family of four, the United States poverty level is set at $23,550 up $2,347 from the 2008 level. Dividing that by twelve months leaves the family with $1880 per month or $60 per day to cover rent, utilities, food, transportation, clothing, and healthcare needs. As HCPs we can easily see that there may be no money left to purchase medication, pay for medical services, or transportation to and from medical appointments.

> *Reflective exercise: Socioeconomic*
> 1. *Have you experienced poverty?*
> 2. *If so, what was your greatest concern?*
> 3. *What are the socioeconomic demographics of your patient population?*
> 4. *How does it compare to your current socioeconomic status?*
> 5. *What are some of the ways you can ensure access to care?*

Health Insurance

Is health insurance the key to wellness? Maybe. Having health insurance makes it possible to seek care, get diagnostic testing, receive physical and/or occupational therapy, get mental health counseling, receive home health visits, and pay for medications. . . . right? Maybe not. Services are dependent on the type of coverage, co-pay requirements and which providers accept your insurance. If finances are an issue, then the choice of coverage is based primarily on cost. For some patients, paying $500 or $1,500 per month for health insurance can be the difference between putting food on the table for their family or going hungry. For the working poor, those who work yet are unable to pay for insurance, the likelihood of securing insurance is questionable.

According to the U.S. Census Bureau, 32% of people are covered by government insurance (Medicare, Medicaid, Military healthcare, State Children's Health Insurance Program and individual state health plans), while 64% are covered by private insurance (plans provided by employers or a union or purchased by an individual from a private company).[5] Healthcare reform continues to be a work in progress, specifically in regard to the cost of drugs, the hospital rates and provider fee.

Let's look specifically at the uninsured from the point of ethnicity, age, and household income. Think about your patient population as you review these statistics posted by the U.S. Census Bureau report, *Income, Poverty and Health Insurance Coverage in the United States: 2012.*

Uninsured by Ethnicity

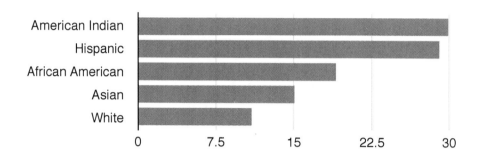

Uninsured by Age

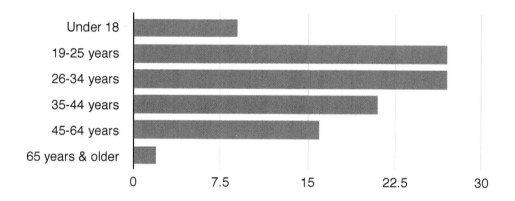

Uninsured by Household Income

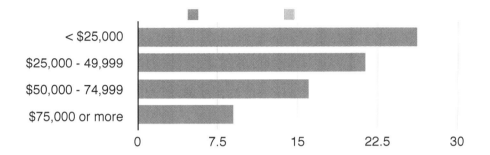

> *Reflective exercise: Health Insurance*
> 1. *Have you ever gone without health insurance?*
> 2. *What change in your life or your finances dictated a decision to forego health insurance?*
> 3. *If so, what was your greatest concern?*
> 4. *Think about your patient population ~ those who are uninsured?*
> 5. *What resources are in place within your organization to meet their health needs?*

Language

Language is how one communicates needs and gains knowledge. Persons not fluent in English may hesitate to seek care unless a translator is available. Numerous studies have shown that those who do not speak English are less likely to receive the same treatment as those who do. According to the *2011 American Community Survey* nearly 21%, or more than fifty million people, speak a language other than English at home. That number has increased over the past decade.

Language Use and English Speaking Ability:2012, issued by the U.S. Census Bureau, indicates that there are more than 381 categories of single languages spoken by persons living in the United States. Those households deemed *linguistically isolated* are defined as those in which no one over the age of 14 speaks English at least "very well." The 2010 census showed an increase in this category from 2.9 million households in 1990 to 4.6 million in 2010.

Those who speak English "less than well" continue to live predominately in Florida, California, New York and Texas followed by states in the Midwest. Yet, as HCPs, we know that statistics are just that – statistics – and may not reflect your site. Lack of bilingual/bicultural HCPs may be perceived by your patients as a barrier to care.

Speakers of Language Other Than English at Home

& English Ability by Language Group

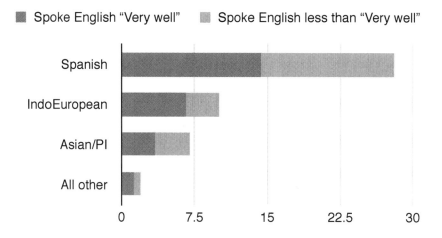

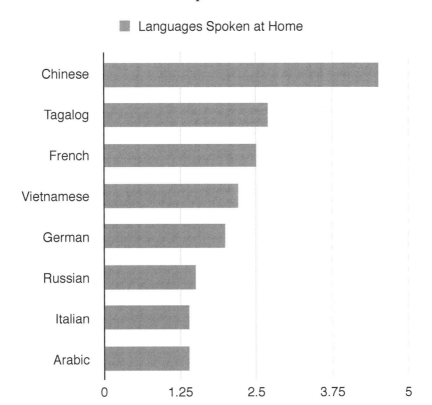

Languages Most Frequently Spoken at Home Other Than English and Spanish

Source: U.S. Census Bureau, Census 2012

Lost in translation . . . ?

English language proficiency is an indicator many use to determine if an immigrant has truly assimilated to the *American culture*. Consider newly arrived immigrant or perhaps those who have been in this country for decades. Their limited English proficiency is viewed in a negative context. In a poll conducted by the Pew Research Center in 2006, 44% of Americans believed that the immigrants of today are not as willing to assimilate as those who came in the early 20th century. In the article, *Engine of Assimilation – the Economy* (2008), Tomas Jimenez, assistant professor of sociology at UC San Diego, counters that assimilation is not a choice, but rather has a direct relationship with educational and economic opportunities. As HCPs who care for multi-ethnic and multi-generational populations, we must acknowledge that assimilation is a process and that language is only one indicator.

As HCPs we face this challenge of language on a daily basis. Ideally, there are health professionals on staff within the organization who speak the patient's language and understand the culture. However, we frequently rely on nonprofessional staff or family members to translate. In either case, unless an interpreter training program is in place, there is minimal assurance that medical information is translated effectively to the patient. Furthermore, asking a family member to translate does not always ensure accuracy. The patient may not share information pertinent to their case because they do not want the family to know personal issues. The HCP, in turn, may not get the whole story.

There are some basic principles to follow when using an interpreter. First, you should meet with the interpreter prior to the encounter and discuss the information you need to share with the patient. It is vital that the entire response made by the patient is given. The following example exemplifies the importance of interpreting all the information shared. A question is asked of the patient, "What time do you take your medication each day?" The response may go on for several minutes, after which time the interpreter says to you, "about 7:00 p.m." Two thoughts emerge – one from you and one from the patient. The patient may think that the interpreter did not tell the whole story, thus trust could become an issue. The HCP may come to the same conclusion – what information was not shared? For many cultural groups, it is in "sharing the story," that the message is encoded. The patient may have shared that she gets up in the morning, does not take the medication because it upsets her stomach and makes her dizzy, and that is why she waits until the end of the day. A person trained in medical translation would acknowledge the importance of that information and provide the HCP with the whole story.

Beyond words, messages are communicated through body language and tone of voice. According to Dr. Mehrabin (1969), 55% of what we say is body language, 38% is tone of voice, and only 7% is words. Here are some additional suggestions to ensure understanding. First, always look at the patient when asking the question, and continue to observe during the translation period. What is her body language and tone of voice saying? Think about the community you serve and the languages spoken. What resources are available to you to learn another language? Are classes offered through your community college or within your organization? An additional resource is immersion programs. These programs are found in many different countries and offer daily language classes and housing with a host family. Language skills and cultural knowledge are the dividends of immersion programs. An even greater reward is the smile on your patient's face when you speak and they understand.

> *Reflective exercise: Language & Communication*
> 1. *Have you ever gotten ill and sought medical care in a country in which you did not speak the language?*
> 2. *If so, how did you communicate your concerns to the HCP?*
> 3. *Did you receive the care and reassurance you were seeking?*
> 4. *Reflect on your healthcare facility ~ What languages are spoken?*
> 5. *Are there bilingual/bicultural HCPs available?*
> 6. *Other translation services?*
> 7. *Does the organization provide funds to educate and certify translators?*

Education & Literacy level

The key to reaching across the divide between HCP and patient, in addition to communication skills, is education and the patient's ability to read and understand handouts. Literacy, defined as the ability to read and write, may not correlate with a patient's educational level. According to the National Assessment of Adult Literacy Figure 6-2 Health Literacy(NAAL) report of 2009, more that 14% or eight million persons in the United States cannot read the label: *"Keep out of reach of children!"* That's eye opening!

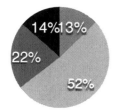

Figure 6-2 Health Literacy

Proficient: can perform complex literacy activities
Intermediate: can perform moderate challenging literacy activities
Basic: can perform simple everyday tasks
Below basic: can perform no more than the simplest and concrete literacy activity.

The National Assessment of Adult Literacy indicates that White and Asian/Pacific Islander adults have a higher health literacy level than Black, Hispanic, American Indian/Alaskan Native and multiracial adults. Reflect for a moment on the educational material available within in your department. Do they match your patient's literacy level?

Health education material, according to *The Institute of Medicine of the National Academics Health Literacy* (2004), is generally written at the eighth grade level. Hospital consent forms are written at a college level. For a large number of persons residing in the United States who are at basic and below level of literacy, it may be a daunting task to read and understand the contents. Health education material should reflect the population of the community and take into account the education and literacy level and the culture.

Here are some suggestions you may want to consider

- Written material should have large amounts of white space so as to appear uncluttered, have large type set (12 point font or more) and good illustrations that reflect the written information.

- Age, gender and culture must be considered in the design of the material.

- Translation of the material into another language takes additional focus requiring two or more native speakers to back-translate the material to ensure understanding.

- Clip art needs to be sensitive to the cultural group as well.

- Personalize the information by using the word "you."

- Medical terminology that would not be understood by the patient should be avoided.

- The document should have good readability.

Another tool for establishing rapport & trust

Neurolinguistic Programming (NLP) is an excellent way to eliminate barriers, establish rapport, and build trust. It is a style of communication based on the way we take in information, encode it, and use it to convey our messages. Information is received through our five senses: sight, sound, feeling, smell, and taste. One or two of these are usually dominant. For example, if you were describing a parade and you encode using sight, your response would include color, float design and costumes worn by the participants. If auditory, you would talk about the sounds you heard. Listen to your patient's words as they tell you about their current health concern. Are they visual, auditory, feeling, taste, or smell? If your patient is an auditory person, you would ask "what *sound* did you hear when you twisted your ankle?" In this way the patient describes the health issue the way she encodes information. As you listen, notice their body stance – where they place their hands, arms and legs – are they leaning in or out. Copying their stand with your own actually brings an intuitive understanding of their concerns and helps to establish trust and rapport. In the book *Maisie Dobbs*, author Jacqueline Winspear describes a scene in which Maisie, private detective in England at the turn of the century, mirrors Celia's (suspect) stance. "*Maisie observed Celia, and once again moved her body to mirror the woman's position. Her head seemed to sink lower on her long neck, her shoulders rounded, her hands tightened with pain. Such melancholy."* Mirroring body language is useful to gather information and understanding the emotional status of the individual.

> *Reflective exercise: Education and Literacy*
> 1. *What is the literacy level of your patient population?*
> 2. *Does your educational material match the literacy level of your patients?*
>   a. *Does it reflect their ethnicity and culture?*
> 3. *What are their options for learning?*
> 4. *Are your educational classes offered in the evening? On the weekend? At the local church? Or a neighborhood school?*

Acculturation and Language

There are a variety of viewpoints and strong opinions about immigrants learning English and assimilating into the American culture. Acculturation or assimilation may factor into one's ability to access healthcare. In a poll conducted by the Pew Research Center in 2006, 44% of Americans believed that the immigrants of today are not as willing to assimilate as those who came in the early 20th century. For some this may be true. Acculturation may be the first thought and focus of a new immigrant or may not occur until the second or third generation. Again we must consider that assimilation has a direct relationship with the economic and educational opportunities.

As HCPs who care for multi-ethnic and multi-generational populations, we need to view each person as a unique individual and not categorize them based on a perceived level of assimilation to this country. Remember how it feels to be new . . . the new employee. . . the new student, or the new kid in the neighborhood? All things are uncomfortable and uncertain. Consider the newly arrived immigrants and those who have lived here for twenty years. Think of ways you can promote understanding, and to create a welcoming environment.

Bilingual & Bicultural

You walk into the hospital or clinic or outpatient therapy department – does anyone working there look like you or talk like you? If the answer is yes, then there is a sense of familiarity and assurance. But what if no one matches you? Would you still feel that level of comfort and familiarity? Perhaps not. Think about your patient population and your staff population. Do they match? And really, is it important? In one study involving African American and white providers, it was noted that the trust level between the patient and the providers was less than that of the other groups.

Current demographics show an increase in ethnic diversity of nurses, social workers, and physicians over the past decade. Given that the U.S. population is significantly more diverse than HCPs, outreach programs that encourage minority students to enter into the healthcare profession are vital. This concept is recognized by many in the health profession, in academia, and in the United States Congress. *Closing the Health Care Gap Act 2004*, as previously mentioned in Chapter 3 Demographics, identified educational and recruitment of minority groups as essential to the elimination of barriers to care and increased access to care. Here are their recommendations.

Professional Education, Awareness and Training

- Workforce Diversity and Training
    - ☐ Increase underrepresented minority students and faculty
    - ☐ Provide funds for scholarships
    - ☐ Increase individuals from disadvantaged backgrounds

- Increase flexibility for use of Higher Education Act funds for historically Black Graduate Institutions

- Model Cultural Competency Curriculum Development

- ☐ Demonstrate series to test models curricula
- ☐ Identify barriers to culturally appropriate care
- ☐ Implement an on-line library with clinically relevant cultural information

The 2002 report by the IOM, *Unequal Treatment: What Health Care System Administrators Need to Know about Racial and Ethnic Disparities in Healthcare*, suggests that both patient and HCPs could benefit from culturally appropriate education. Providing on-site cultural awareness education seminars for staff increases the cultural knowledge and skills to provide culturally competent healthcare to a diverse population. Providing patients with information about ways to access healthcare, to participate in the decision-making process, and to navigate the healthcare system may increase their confidence to advocate for their needs. Together with our patients we can address issues and work collaboratively to eliminate the barriers to healthcare.

Resources

Armstrong, K., Ravenell, K.L., McMurphy, S., Putt, M. (2007). Racial/Ethnic differences in physician distrust in the United States. *American Journal of Public Health.* 97(7). pp. 1283-1289.

Andrews, M., Boyle, J. (2008). *Transcultural concepts in nursing care.* (5th Ed.). New York: Wolters Kluwer

Campinha-Bacote, J. (2003). *The process of cultural competence in the delivery of healthcare services: A culturally competent model of care.* Cincinnati, OH: Transcultural C.A.R.E. Associates.

Farrell, C. (2006). It's time to cure health care. *Business Week.* www.businessweek.com

Giger, J. (2013). *Transcultural nursing: Assessment and intervention.* (6th Ed.). New York: Elsevier Mosby.

Giger, J., Davidhizar, R., Purnell, L., Harden, J., Phillips, J., Stickland. (2007).American Academy of Nursing Expert Panel Report: Developing cultural competence to eliminate health disparities in ethnic minorities and other vulnerable populations. *Journal of Transcultural Nursing.* (18) 2, 95-102.

Hoffman, B. (2003). Health Care Reform and Social Movements in the United States. *American Journal of Public Health.* (93)1. 75-85.

Institute of Medicine of the National Academics. (2004). Health Literacy: A prescription to end confusion. Retrieved on July 9, 2009from www.iom/edu

Jimenez, T. (2008). Engine of assimilation–the economy. *San Francisco Chronicle.*

Kaiser Family Foundation. (2009). Focus on health reform: Side by side comparison major health care reform proposals.

Krogstad, J.M. (2014). One in Four Native Americans and Alaskan Native Living in Poverty. RetrievedSeptember 22, 2015 from pewresearch.org

Leininger, M., McFarland, M. (2002). *Transcultural nursing: Concepts, theories, research and practice.* (3rd Ed.). New York: McGraw-Hill.

Lincoln, B. (2010). *Reflections from Common Ground: Cultural Awareness in Healthcare.* Wisconsin: PesiHealthcare

Lipson, J., Dibble, S., Minarik, P. (2001). *Culture & Nursing Care: A pocket guide*. San Francisco: UCSF Nursing Press,

McGoldrick, M., Giordano, J., Garcia-Preto, N. (2005). *Ethnicity and family therapy.* (3rd Ed). New York: Guilford Press.

Mehrabin, A. Mehrabin Communication Study 1969. Retrieved November 3, 2009, from www.kaaj/com/psych

Murray, C., Woods, V.D. (2009). Psychology of Health Disparities among African American populations: An overview. *Journal of Black Psychology.* (35)2, 142-145,

Purnell, L.D. (2013). *Transcultural health care: A culturally competent approach.* (4th Ed.). Philadelphia, PA: F.A. Davis Company.

Sandoval, V., Adams, S. (2001). Subtle skills for building rapport using neuro-linguistic programming in the interview room. *FBI Law Enforcement Bulletin* 1-5.

Siatkowshi, A. (2007). Hispanic acculturation: A concept analysis. *Journal of Transcultural Nursing.* (18)4, 316-323.

Smedley, B., Stith, A., Nelson, A. (2002). Unequal treatment: Confronting racial and ethnic disparities in health care. Institute of Medicine. Washington D.C.: The National Academies Press.

Spector, R. (2012). *Cultural diversity in health and illness.* (8th Ed.), New Jersey: Pearson/Prentice Hall.

Villarruel, A. (2007). Poverty and health disparities: More than just a difference. *Western Journal of Nursing Research.* (29)6, 654-656.

Wooley, J., Peters, G. (2009). *The American Presidency Report.* University of California: Santa Barbara.

University of Kentucky. (2009). Cross-Cultural Communication. Office of Student Activities, Leadership & Involvement. www.uky.edu/studentactivities/leadership

U.S. Department of Commerce. (2012). Language use and English-speaking ability: 2010. U.S. Census Bureau. Economics and Statistics Administration. U.S.

U.S. Department of Commerce. Denavas-Walt, C., Proctor, B.D., Smith, J.C. (2012). Income, Poverty, and Health Insurance Coverage in the United States: 2012,

US Department of Commerce. Ryan, C. (2013). Language Use in the United States: 2011. American Community Survey Reports

Department of Education. (2010). A first look at the literacy of America's adults in the 21st century. National Center for Educational Statistics.

U.S. Department of Social Security. (2009). Social Insurance Movement. Retrieved March 8, 2010, from www.socialsecurity.gov/history.

Finding Common Ground | 6

"Culture is a mediator between human beings and chaos, guiding our interactions with each other." – *Julie Lipson 1996*

The road to cultural competence begins with "aha" moments of discovery. We suddenly and unexpectedly grasp an understanding of our cultural – beliefs, values, and biases – the way each guides our interactions and influences our decisions. During these moments we realize our similarities and differences with patients and colleagues. Our willingness to meet and honor those who may be different from us is the beginning of cultural competence. Stops along the way open the door to finding common ground, understanding and respect.

Cultural beliefs and values ~ First Stop

Culture – we all have it! It is how we reveal ourselves to others. We may not realize its influence because it is so embedded that we take it for granted. However, others see us differently. Why? Because they view us through their cultural lenses. For those of us working with multi-ethnic communities this could pose a significant dilemma, as our culture may be different than theirs. So how do we bridge this potential barrier? Initially we can start with understanding and valuing each other's culture.

Culture can be defined as beliefs and values passed down from one generation to the next. Think back to your family of origin. What were the important beliefs and values in your family? Perhaps they were values such as respect, work hard, educational achievement, financial stability, and telling the truth? Here are some other questions to consider. How were decisions made? What were the views on education and economics? How did religion influence your family's healthcare practices? Now, what happens when your list does not match that of your patient or your colleague? Conflict? Misunderstanding? We do well not to take it personally, but rather to understand that each person is seeing through his or her cultural filters. The following exercise is an opportunity to discover your cultural values and beliefs.

> *Reflective exercise: Cultural beliefs and values*
> 1. *List two beliefs you learned as a child.*
> 2. *Who did you learn them from?*
> 3. *Are they still important to you today?*
> 4. *Have you experienced conflict when your values/beliefs did not match those of another?*
> 5. *Where do you find common ground with patients and colleagues?*

Were you surprised by your reponses? These values and beliefs are unique to *"your story."* You rely on them in times of uncertainty. Julie Lipson (1996), researcher and educator, captures this concept in her definition of culture. For her, culture is "the mediator between human beings and chaos, guiding our interactions with each other" (p.1). As those of us in the field know that healthcare settings can be stressful, our cultural values and beliefs provide the support and confidence needed to grapple with the chaos.

Next Stop ~ Cultural Awareness

The next step in the journey to cultural competence begins with cultural awareness: an opportunity to acknowledge, appreciate, and accept one's cultural values, beliefs and to recognize biases learned as a child. These "aha" moments of discovery broaden our world view and help us to find common ground with patients and colleagues. We know that conflict occurs when our beliefs and values are in direct contrast with others. Differences, once considered barriers, can now give way to bridges of understanding and respect. Think about people and groups that are not part of *your every day*. Are there biases or assumption you have about them?

> *Reflective exercise: Cultural Awareness*
> 1. *What ethnic, religious, political or generational group do you associate with on a regular basis?*
> 2. *Reflect on some encounter you had with those who are members of a different or opposing group.*
> 3. *Did you recognize any biases or prejudices toward that person?*
> 4. *How did that feel?*

When we encounter people different from ourselves, we have the opportunity to gain insight into their world. The more opportunities we pursue, the more enlightened we become. Cultural awareness education seminars, field trips, language immersion programs and case presentations are venues that help to increase cultural awareness. Wade Davis, Ethnobiologist, said it well. "The world in which you were born is just one model of reality. Other cultures are not failed attempts at being you: they are unique manifestations of the human spirit." Cultural humility, the next step on the journey, challenges us to pause, reflect and be open to another's perspective.

We're getting there ~ the next stop ~ Cultural Humility

What is cultural humility? According to Tervalon and Murray-Garcia who first coined the phrase, "it is an ongoing process of self-reflection and self-critique, a way of being aware of our relationship with others and ourselves (1997 p.117)." It is not static. Cultural humility encourages us not only to recognize and acknowledge our biased assumptions, but to take responsibility for our actions/interactions with others. It calls us to identify power inequities that may exist between us and our patients.

> *Reflective exercise: Cultural Humility Case Scenario*
> *You are admitting an elderly, limited English speaking woman to your medical unit. She is alone. She has poor dental hygiene, wears mismatched clothes and smells badly.*
> 1. *What are you immediate thoughts?*
> 2. *Name one or more biases that spontaneously come to mind.*
> 3. *Understanding the concept of cultural humility – how would you approach her?*

Awareness brings about humility, which brings further awareness, and ultimately, a change in the way we approach each encounter. Seeing through the eyes of another helps us to discover common ground, enabling us to develop respectful partnerships that are patient centered. We are now ready for the final stage of the journey, cultural competence.

Cultural Competence

Cultural competence is an ongoing process. It begins with an inner desire to know more about other cultures and a willingness to encounter the uncomfortable. Cultural knowledge is acquired with each encounter and every discussion. It summons us to think outside of our "cultural world." Gaining awareness, knowledge and skill leads to heightened cultural sensitivity and competence. Are your ready?

> *Reflective exercise: Cultural Competence*
> 1. *What is motivating me to become culturally competent?*
> 2. *What do I want/need to know about other cultures ... and where do I find this information?*
> 3. *When I experience cultural encounters, how does it feel and what do I learn?*
> 4. *Whom do I consider a "cultural resource person" in my life?*

Cultural Assessments . . . Planning Care

In order to provide a cultural assessment, three elements are necessary. First, we must be aware of our cultural beliefs, values, biases and healthcare practices; second, we must have the knowledge of various ethnic groups; and third, we must have the practical skills necessary to complete a cultural assessment.

In this section we review each of the elements in the author's model Reflections from Common Ground (Figure 6-1). This model provides an opportunity to discover your culture and then identify similarities and differences with patients and colleagues. Here you will find common ground that lays the foundation for providing culturally sensitive and competent care. As you review each element, ask yourself, "How am I the same or different from my patient and where do I find common ground?"

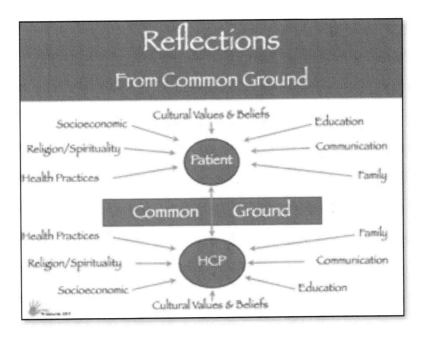

Figure 6.1 Reflections from Common Ground

Our Words . . . Our ways of Communicating

Communication, verbal and non verbal, is an expression of ourselves – how we reveal ourselves to others. It is our response to encounters with life. Think about your style of communication as you do the next reflective exercise.

> *Reflective exercise: Communication*
> 1. *Do I speak loudly or softly?*
> 2. *Do I speak quickly or slowly?*
> 3. *Does the tone of my voice match my words . . . my message?*
> 4. *Does my body language match my words . . . my message?*
> 5. *Do I use facial expressions & gestures to convey my message?*
> 6. *Is eye contact important to my conversation or do I consider it intrusive?*
> 7. *Is touch an acceptable element of my conversation*
> 8. *Silence – Am I uncomfortable with long period of silence? Do I use it when I do not want to create conflicts or I do not agree with another? It is part of my style?*

Now that you have identified your style of communication, think about your family of origin. Do you see similarities? My guess is that you have heard people comment, "You sound just like your mom . . . your dad . . . your sister . . .brother." Your style is reflective of your life. It's comfortable and fits you perfectly!

The next question to ask yourself – how is my style similar to or different from my patients' and colleagues. Do I feel a disconnect when it seems my message is not getting across. We know from "Communication 101" the more we reflect the tone, speed, voice quality and stance of our patient, the more information we receive. This reflective technique breaks down barriers, builds rapport and establishes trust. Caution must be taken not to form an opinion about another's unique style of communication; it is just different. Robert Williams, educator and researcher, sums it up well. "My language is me. It is an extension of my being, my essence. It is a reflection and badge of my culture. Criticism of my language is essentially a direct attack on my self esteem and cultural identity." [6]

Time . . . How we use it!

Time orientation may be an issue when you are a "to be early is to be on time person" and your patient/colleague is a "get there when I do" person. Time orientation can be viewed from the perspective of seasonal change, the rhythms of social life, and clock time. In this section we will focus on time as past, present, future orientation. While we use all three, two dominate. How we interpret and use time is culturally learned. In the following exercise, please read all six statements, and then choose two that closely reflect your view of time.

> *Reflective exercise: My use of time*
> 1. *My ancestors protect and guide me*
> 2. *To be early is to be on time*
> 3. *Can't we go back to the way it use to be!*
> 4. *Here and now – Carpe diem!*
> 5. *Planning for the future is hopeless*
> 6. *I have planned for my retirement*

If you are past oriented then respect and honor for the elderly and ancestors in your family/community are important. You seek out their knowledge and wisdom. Resistance to change falls into this category as well. The phrase "can't we go back to the way it use to be" conveys a value for past events in contrast with the current situation. It is difficult to transition into the new way of doing things. Another frequently heard phrase, "Remember the good old days," offers familiarity and security. Change may cause stress and anxiety. Yet, if given an opportunity to participate in the process of change, you may be more likely to be accepting of the outcome.

Present day orientation focuses on today, thus planning for the future may seem futile. "Here and now" feels more comfortable and safe. Your attention to the immediate needs of a patient, colleague, or family member supersedes punctuality. Unfortunately, this may cause others to see you as disorganized in the work setting. Caring for a patient, or taking time to help a colleague ensures that you're meeting their needs.

If you are future oriented, "to be early is to be on time" resonates closely with your thinking. It's all about the future! Vacations are scheduled well in advance. You are motivated to plan for the future by getting a college degree that translates into a better paying job and a secure future. You set timelines to achieve long-term goals. In the workplace you are lauded for your ability to organize your time, set priorities and get work done on time.

It is essential that we understand that our view of time may be different from others. Working with a patient or a colleague to determine the best approach helps to assure understanding and respect for differences.

> *Reflective exercise: Time*
> 1. *How are you different from you patient population?*
> 2. *Where do you find common ground?*

My Space ~ don't come too close!

Spatial orientation is a learned value. From an early age you were taught, usually tacitly, the appropriate distance between you and family, friends and outsiders. At home, or with extended family, you may be "up close and personal," but this may not translate into acceptable behavior in public. Using what is considered the appropriate space in one situation may not be viewed as respectful in another. Have you had the experience of persons invading your "personal space," assuming a familiarity that didn't exist? For them it may just be "who they are." They find it surprising that you are annoyed.

Space, in Western culture, offers three dimensions: intimate, personal, and public. Intimate space, designated as zero to eighteen inches, is used by close friends and family. Personal space, eighteen inches to three feet, is used by friends, acquaintances, some colleagues, counselors, and family members. Three to six feet, public space, is used when conducting interviews or business transactions. Other cultural groups may use different parameters. Observing patients' use of space before assuming differently.

> *Reflective exercise: Spatial orientation*
> 1. *When you are talking with close friends and family, how much distance is between you?*
> 2. *Does gender or age determine space?*
> 3. *How do you react when someone "invades" your personal space?*
> 4. *How are you different from your patients or colleagues?*
> 5. *Where do you find common ground?*

Family

The definition of family today is different than fifty or even twenty years ago. The U.S. Census Bureau defines *family* as "people who occupy the same house." Webster's definition relates to the "descendants from a common progenitor, a tribe, clan, or race." While definitions vary, we do know that families have a significant influence in the development of cultural beliefs, values, and health practices. They provide a social framework that is internalized and accepted as normative and true.

Married with no children, two parent families with children, extended family, single parent, blended, alternative and same sex partners are all considered, by definition, to be family. Within each of these family structures are assigned roles and responsibilities. Each designates status and duty. Defined roles provide the support necessary to to maintain family harmony during an illness. We know that dynamics of a family can change with the diagnosis of stroke, heart attack, cancer or diabetes. Who now assumes the role of decision maker and caregiver when a member can no longer fulfill his or her role? What is the response from other members of the family to the change?

Conflict may arise when your view of family responsibilities and roles does not match those of your patient population. For example, suppose you were raised in a two-parent family that espoused an egalitarian view, but your patient comes from a patriarchal family with clearly defined gender roles. Expectations are different. During times of uncertainty for your patient, you can show support and respect by acknowledging differences and working collaboratively with the patient to develop a plan of care that incorporates the cultural values and beliefs about family.

> *Reflective exercise: Family*
> 1. *What was the structure of your family when you were growing up?*
> 2. *What was your role and responsibility?*
> 3. *Who was the decision maker?*
> 4. *What was the role of the sick person?*
> 5. *What is the structure of your current family? Is it the same or different from that of your family of origin?*
> 6. *How are you different from your patient population?*
> 7. *Where do you find common ground?*
> 8. *Where do you find common ground?*

Religion/Spirituality

Religion and spirituality may be a source of comfort during difficult times. Religion, thought of as an organized group structure, offers comfort through its set of beliefs and practices based on the teachings of a spiritual icon or leader such as Jesus, Buddha, Mohammed or Brigham Young. The Bible, Torah, Qu'ran, the Book of Mormon, and other holy texts provide the written word which, when followed, offer a source of well-being and enlightenment. Spirituality take a more individualistic approach. It is thought of as a journey in which one seeks awareness and personal meaning from each experience. This translates to an awareness of one's purpose of life. Heightened spirituality, as with religion, offers a sense of support and hope during times of uncertainty. Both provide a supportive foundation when facing a diagnosis of terminal cancer, a colleague's diagnosis of multiple sclerosis, a spouse with end stage symptoms of Huntington's chorea, or a nephew coping with schizophrenia.

There are hundreds of organized religions in the United States. Each hold strong beliefs about health, illness and cure. Adherence to the religious beliefs and practices for some equates to health and harmony. For others, illness is seen as a punishment from God or as a result of failure to follow religious tenets. For one of my patients this was her reality. She stated assuredly that "God made her bedridden so she would stop what she was doing and listen." The cause of her illness was based on her religious beliefs, and healing would come when she was obedient to God.

Recognizing the importance of religion and spirituality, hospitals across the country have added pastoral care departments. They provide support to patients and families from varied religious affiliations. Together with the patient and pastoral care you can develop a plan of care that acknowledges and incorporates religious and spiritual beliefs.

> *Reflective exercise: Religion & Spirituality*
> 1. *As a child were you part of a religious denomination? . . . Is it the same today?*
> 2. *Is spirituality an influence in your life?*
> 3. *In what ways do religion and/or spirituality affect your health? Illness?*
> 4. *How do your beliefs of religion/spirituality contrast with those of your patient population?*
> 5. *Where do you find common ground?*

Education . . .

Education, whether from institutions or life experiences, lays a foundation that influences how we learn. We acquire tools that enable us to take in, process, and use new information.

> *Reflective exercise: Education*
> 1. *How do you learn best? Narrative, Written, Hands On?*
> 2. *How many years of schooling do you have?*
> 3. *How does your education and learning style different from your patient population?*
> 4. *Where do you find common ground?*

When you think of your patients, the most important question to ask is "how do you learn best?" rather than "how far did you go in school?" The stigma attached to those who have less than a high school education may prejudice your perspective of the patient's abilities. The patient's ability to read, write, and comprehend information must be assessed. More importantly, though, is the method of learning that is most effective for each person. Your patients may learn by watching videos, participating in a demonstration to learn a technique or engaging in group discussion. Or, they may choose to combine all three methods.

Socioeconomics

How your family used money for healthcare in the past may influence how you use it now. Phrases like "we don't go to the doctor unless it is absolutely necessary," or "if I go to the hospital, I'll never come home again," may influence the decision to seek healthcare. One's socioeconomic status affects how finances are managed and dictates decisions about healthcare. It is prudent for you to be knowledgeable about available resources for patients and to create an environment that promotes dignity and respect for those whose finances may be a barrier to care.

Healthcare practices

Your definition of health and illness also influences the decision to seek professional care or rely on folk practices and proven "home remedies." Professional care, we know, focuses on the biological cause and treatment of an illness, which may include medicine or surgery. Folk care factors in home remedies passed down from one generation to the next. You may have been the recipient of some of these remedies as a child – Vick's® VapoRub® on the chest for a cold, ginger ale and soda crackers for nausea, and carrot syrup for a cough. Many believe that healing can occur using both approaches – professional and folk.

Included in healthcare beliefs is one's ability or lack of ability to control their health status. Locus of control can be viewed as internal or external. An internal locus of control suggests that you have the ability to control a situation and to influence the outcome. So, if you follow the plan, eat well, exercise and get enough sleep, then health is ensured. In contrast, when you ascribe to an external locus of control, efforts and reward are not related. You health is the result of luck, chance or faith.

> *Reflective exercise: Health Practices*
> 1. *Is your primary approach to healthcare – professional? folk? or both?*
> 2. *Do you have an internal or external locus of control?*
> 3. *How do you contrast with those in your patient population?*
> 4. *Where do you find common ground?*

It is important to note the patient's definition of health and illness and the locus of control when inquiring about their cultural health practices and beliefs. This topic will be addressed in greater detail in Chapter 7, *Ancient wisdom...Modern medicine,* as well as in the vignettes.

Ancient wisdom, folk care practices, and healers are still an integral part of many of our patients. The combination of the two modalities for some is the key to recovery. Knowledge of our patient's cultural health practices leads to understanding, acceptance and respect for differences. The goal is to provide quality care that integrates cultural beliefs and values into the plan of care. Culturally competent care is the result of both cultural awareness and knowledge. An inquisitive HCP seeks out information from the patient to assure that all possibilities have been uncovered. Together you develop a plan of care that incorporates cultural beliefs, values and health practices into the healing process.

Developing a Plan of Care - Culture Care Decisions & Actions

In each of the preceding sections we gained patient information. These responses are deeply embedded in one's belief system. Our mission is to listen, learn, and respect their cultural beliefs and values. During these discussions we consider the impact – positive or negative – on their healthcare decisions and practices. The following three modes of care decisions and actions guide us in the development of a plan of care. These include acknowledgement, adjustment, and change.

Acknowledge and Affirm values the beliefs and health practices of the patient. Acknowledging the support given the patients by the inclusion into the plan of care demonstrates a genuine understanding by the HCP of their importance in care. These practices might include:

- *A string tied around wrist or ankle to protect wellbeing*
- *Respect for the elderly*
- *Avoiding eye contact and not raising one's voice*
- *Praying five times each day*
- *Visits by a priest, monks, an imam, church elders, deacons*

Discuss and Adjust assures the patient that the HCP understands these values and makes adjustments in the plan of care to incorporate them. Recognizing the significance of the cultural values, and including them in the plan, demonstrates awareness and respect on the part of the HCP.

- *Family participation in care*
- *Obligation and expectation to visit the sick ~ flexible visiting hours*
- *Kosher meals for the Orthodox Jewish patient*
- *Ceremonies/rituals in the hospital room for the dying patient*
- *Overnight accommodation for a parent to stay with a child*

Change may be necessary when a patient's current health practices are detrimental to their health and wellbeing. While this discussion may cause tension between the HCP and the patient, it is an opportunity that leads to a greater understanding. **Collaborating** in a respectful manner opens doors to creative solutions. Areas where conflict might arise include concepts such as:

- *Avoiding surgery until the full moon*
- *Taking medication only when symptoms are present ~ HTN, NIDM*
- *Eating large amounts of rice ~ a diabetic patient*
- *Sedentary lifestyle in an obese patient*
- *Eating for two ~ pregnant woman with gestational diabetes*

In this chapter we determined that cultural competency is a journey and that it begins with self-awareness. The reflective exercises provided you with an opportunity to discover your cultural beliefs, values, biases and healthcare practices and contrast them with those of patients and colleagues. It is through this process that you find common ground and build the bridge to understanding. Creating an environment that promotes dignity, respect and openness to other perspectives increases rapport and helps ensure a trusting relationships.

Resources

Andrews, M. M., Boyle, J. S. (2008). *Transcultural concepts in nursing care.* (5th Ed.). New York: Wolters Kluwer.
Campinha-Bacote, J. (2003). *The process of cultural competence in the delivery of healthcare services: A culturally competent model of care.* Cincinnati, OH: Transcultural C.A.R.E. Associates
Gay, G. (2004). *Culturally responsive teaching: Theory, research & practice.* New York: Teachers College Press.
Giger, J. N. (2013). *Transcultural nursing: Assessment and intervention.* (6th Ed.). St Louis, MO: Mosby/Elsevier.
Leininger, M. M. (1991). *Culture care diversity and universality: A theory of nursing.* New York: National League for Nursing Press.
Leininger, M. M., McFarland, M. R. (2002). *Transcultural nursing: Concepts, theories, research and practice.* (3rd Ed.). New York: McGraw-Hill.
Lincoln, B. (2010). *Reflections from Common Ground: Cultural Awareness in Healthcare.* Wisconsin: PesiHealthcare
McFarland, M.R., Wehbe-Alamah, H. (2014). *Culture Care Diversity and Universality: A Worldwide Nursing Theory.*
Lipson, J. G., Dibble, S. L., Minarik, P. A. (1996). *Culture & Nursing Care: A pocket guide.* San Francisco: UCSF Nursing Press.
McGoldrick, M., Giordano, J., Garcia-Preto, N (2005). *Ethnicity & Family Therapy.* (3rd Ed.). New York: The Guilford Press.
Payne, R. (1996). *The Framework of Poverty.* (3rd Ed.). Texas: aha! Process, Inc.
Purnell, L. D. (2013). *Transcultural Health Care: A Culturally Competent Approach.* (4th Ed.). Philadelphia, PA: F. A. Davis Company.
Sandoval, V. A., Adams, S. H. (2001). Subtle skills for building rapport using neuro-linguistic programming in the interview room. *FBI Law Enforcement Bulletin* 1-5.
Spector, R. (2012). *Cultural diversity in health and illness.* (8th Ed.), New Jersey: Pearson/Prentice Hall.
Tervalon, M., Murray-Garcia, J. (1997). Cultural humility versus cultural competence: A criticial, distinction in defining physician training outcomes in multicultural education. *Journal of Health Care for the Poor and Underserved.* (9)2, 117-125.

Ancient Wisdom... Modern Medicine | 7

Ancient wisdom, folk care and practices, are passed down from one generation to the next. Healing poultices, coining and cupping (use of heat to remove illness from the body), pinching, massage, herbs, and sweat lodges may be used in the curative process. Professional care, on the other hand, refers to modern medicine taught at colleges and universities. The focus is on physical exams, blood tests, x-rays and ultrasounds to diagnose. Pharmaceuticals and surgery provide the cure. Patients may subscribe to both ancient wisdom and modern medicine depending on circumstances.

Realizing that cultural beliefs and health care practices are part of our patient's world view, it may be advantageous to inquire about his or her thoughts about the cause of the illness. One of my patients presented with upper respiratory symptoms which included congestion and a productive cough for one week. She told me she became ill when she "opened the window too fast and the wind got insider her." I was taken aback by her unexpected statement and paused while pondering an effective and sensitive response. Additional questions demonstrated an interest on my part to know more, thus she was more open to sharing her concerns.

We as HCPs view health, illness, caring, and cure as well-defined concepts within our professional training and education. Our patients, who do not speak our "medical language" may give these concepts different meaning and value. How one perceives and defines health, illness, expectations of behavior and response to treatment is influenced by his or her family of origin.

> *Reflective exercise ... Health & Illness*
> 1. *I know I am healthy when ....*
> 2. *I know I am sick when ...*
> 3. *The role of the sick person in our family is ....*
> 4. *Some of the ways my family shows care when someone is ill ..?*

Responses vary. Our cultural awareness education seminar participants share comments such as "I know that I am healthy when I wake up and feel well," "I feel happy and energetic," "I don't have pain;" or the opposite, "I have pain;" "I'm tired all the time," and "I feel sad." Health or illness can be related to a physical or emotional state or a combination of both.

What was the role of the sick person in your family? Was it his or her job to loll on the couch and have others cater to their every need? Or were they required to "rise above" the illness and to continue to function in spite of the illness? It varies according to culture and traditional health beliefs.

Care can be thought of in terms of the verbs: "to care" and "to give care." As HCPs we must acknowledge that the caring practices of various ethnic groups may differ from our prescribed treatment plan, and this may cause misunderstandings and conflict. Knowledge and incorporation of the patient's cultural beliefs may help bridge the divide we experience with patients.

Health Traditions Model

In her book *Cultural Diversity in Health and Illness,* Dr. Rachel Spector, focuses on health and illness as it relates to cultural traditions and practices of health maintenance, protection, and restoration. Heritage consistency, a theory developed by Estes and Zitow, looks at the extent to which one's life is reflective of his or her culture. Dr. Spector expands that concept to acknowledge the importance of traditional health practices and beliefs. Her definition of heritage consistency, "is a means of identification with a traditional ethnocultural heritage leading to the observance of the health/illness beliefs and practices of one's traditional cultural belief system."[7] She sees it as an interwoven influence of one's culture, religion, ethnicity, and socialization. What are the traditions necessary to maintain, protect and restore health? Taking into consideration acculturation, she posits that the more one identifies with traditional culture, the more likely one is to adhere to the cultural values and practices associated with its beliefs of health and illness.

Dr. Spector's model, HEALTH Traditions focuses on a traditional view of ways to maintain HEALTH, protect HEALTH and to restore HEALTH. To differentiate the definition of health from HEALTH, Spector has written 'health' in a small but capitalized format. HEALTH refers to the balance in interrelatedness of one's physical, mental and spiritual being. The model employs a holistic perspective of the individual or community to discover traditional modes of maintaining, protecting, and restoring health. This information in combination with the HCP's plan of care provides a solid foundation for the continued well-being of the patient.

What factors does one need to consider to maintain health? For some it may be adequate nutritional intake, exercise and rest. For others it may mean, in addition to the aforementioned, good relationships with family and friends. For others, it is a strong religious base with rituals that provide well-being. HEALTH maintenance assures that if the patient adheres closely to those practices that promote a healthy lifestyle, then good health is more secure.

HEALTH protection identifies those activities that would protect one from illness or harm. These may include special food, protective objects, or prayers. In some cultural groups such as the Hmong population, people are encouraged to wear red strings about their wrists to protect them from the Dab (an evil spirit that can cause illness), or Chinese American parents may tape a red envelope under the crib of their newborn infant in the neonatal intensive care unit to ensure health.

HEALTH restoration of body, mind, and spirit is achieved through a variety of means and may include home remedies, massage, prayers, religious rituals, and support from family and community. In the Vietnamese culture, coining and cupping may be used to exorcise the illness from the body in order to restore health. Native American populations often use the sweat lodge to provide the restoration of health, physically and spiritually.

> *Reflective exercise - As you consider the HEALTH Traditions Model . .*
> 1. *How do you maintain your health?*
> 2. *Protect your health?*
> 3. *Restore your health?*
> 4. *How are your responses different from those of your patient population?*

Approaches to Health & Wellness

We cannot be experts on every culture and traditional healing practices. In this section we will focus on three specific approaches, as does Foster in his book *Medical Anthropology*.[8] These are biomedicine, personalistic, and naturalistic. Each offers a distinct focus on the cause of illness, the treatment plan, cure, and preventative measures that can be used to ensure wellness.

Biomedicine Approach

Biomedicine, the dominant belief found in the United States and in Western countries, is viewed from the perspective that illness is a result of "cause and effect." Causes include susceptibility to a virus or a bacteria, poor nutrition, exposure to chemicals, injury, or the aging process. Diagnosis is made through the use of laboratory findings, cultures, and x-rays which corroborate physical findings. Treatments include medication, patient education, and follow-up care. Prevention of illness is contingent on the active participation of the individual. Avoidance of pathogens, recreational drugs, alcohol and high risk behavior are on the list. A healthy diet, regular exercise, adequate rest, and vitamin supplements may be other ways a patient maintains health.

As HCPs, this approach is the most familiar to our repertoire as it is the basis of our educational training: identify the cause, provide a treatment, and cure the illness. Consider our patient with the upper respiratory symptoms. With this biomedicine approach, we inquire as to onset and symptoms, take vital signs; perform a physical assessment, and prescribe an antibiotic or rest and plenty of fluids if the illness is attributed to a viral infection. Simple and straight-forward.

Personalistic Approach

What if this respiratory illness is caused by something outside of that realm? What if supernatural forces are causing health issues of the body, mind, spirit ...what then? The personalistic approach, found in the indigenous populations of the Americas as well as Southeast Asia, assumes that the cause of one's illness is secondary to an affliction caused by something paranormal. The "sick person" is the object of punishment by a supernatural being (deity or god), non human forces (ghost, ancestor or evil spirit) or by a human being (witch, sorcerer).

Illness may occur because certain rituals of respect were not given to the ancestor. Special days such as El Dia de Los Muertos in the Mexican tradition or Sweeping the Tomb found in the Chinese and Vietnamese populations, are annual events that give respect to ancestors. On this day, the family goes to the cemetery and cleans the grave of the deceased. They bring this person's favorite food, share stories about the individual, and recognize the importance of that person in their lives. In the pueblo of Pazquero, Mexico, the community rises at midnight and proceeds en masse to the cemetery carrying candles to light the way. They remain at the site throughout the day. This ritual ensures good relationships with the ancestors who are thought to offer protection against illness.

Some cultures believe that non humans can cause illness as well. In the book, *The Spirit Catches You and You Fall Down*, written by Anne Fadiman,[9] a three month old Hmong child becomes ill after her sister slams the door. The parents believed that her soul had left her body and became lost. The emergency room physician ordered an x-ray and told the parents the child had "bronchopneumonia or tracheobronchitis." He ordered antibiotics – a biomedicine approach. Following the emergency room visit, the family sought out the clan's txiv neb, a Hmong healer. They requested a ceremony which would return the child's soul and thus restore health.

In addition to rituals and healing ceremonies, cures may include offering prayers, lighting candles to lift spells, and visits by clergy. You may also see patients wearing amulets or carrying other protective objects which are thought to ensure health. As HCPs, we need to ask the patient what is needed to restore health. Prevention in the personalistic approach includes maintaining good relationships not only with the living, but also with ancestors and deities.

Naturalistic Approach

Health returns when balance is restored in the naturalistic approach. It is all about balance! This approach to health and illness is found primarily in Asian countries, Latin America and in the Philippines. The cause of an illness is an exposure to excessive hot or cold, creating an imbalance which leads to illness. Whether a illness is deemed hot or cold is based on the health beliefs and practices of the individual or group.

Treatment comes in the form of balancing a hot condition with a cold solution and vice versa. It may be helpful to ask about what the patient believes is needed to restore balance. If a hospitalized patient is refusing certain foods or medicines, that may be our cue to inquire if other foods (deemed hot or cold) would be appreciated. Prevention is assured with one's ability to maintain the balance of mind, body, and spirit. Eating the right foods, getting enough rest, and avoiding disagreements with family and friends may indeed ensure a more healthy life.

These three approaches, biomedicine, personalistic and naturalistic may coexist with one another. While in Western countries, biomedicine is dominant, other treatment modalities may also be applied. We may not be aware of it; we need to ask.

Locus of control is an important variable that must be considered in order to plan care that is effective and consistent with the patient's beliefs and practices. People with an internal locus of control believe in their ability to control the environment, thus protecting their health. The belief of adherence to a healthy lifestyle, which includes annual physical exams, good nutritional intake, and daily exercise, ensures a healthy life.

Those with an external locus of control believe that they do not have the power or ability to effect maintenance of health. Fate, luck, chance and God are the controllers. This sometimes is referred to as a "fatalistic" approach – always thinking the worst. As a HCP you may hear someone say "If it is God's will," thus and such will happen, inferring health maintenance is out of his or her control. The patient may not be interested in wellness programs, stop smoking programs, or exercise regimes that are suggested. As HCP's, we can acknowledge the patient's belief, and share some internal locus of control methods that may enable the patient to see positive outcomes and renewed sense of well-being.

> *Reflective exercise ~ Health Beliefs & Practices*
> 1. *My approach to health is usually*
>   *Biomedicine...Personalistic...Naturalistic?*
> 2. *My patient population is usually?*
> 3. *My locus of control is internal or external?*
> 4. *My patient population locus of control?*

It's All About Balance

Four Humors . . . Hot/Cold . . . Yin/Yang . . . Wind

Four Humors ~ Hot & Cold Theory

How does one restore balance or better yet, maintain balance? The Four Humors (Figure 7-3) date back to the beginning of the second century when Hippocrates, a Greek physician, first coined the term. These four elements, considered ether-like qualities emanating from the brain, balance the body to prevent illness from entering. This theory of existed even into the 19th century.

Element	Body	Temperature	Moisture	Personality	Season
Air	**Blood**	Hot	Wet	Sanguine	Spring
Fire	**Yellow Bile**	Hot	Dry	Choleric	Summer
Water	**Phlegm**	Cold	Wet	Phlegmatic	Winter
Earth	**Black Bile**	Cold	Dry	Melancholic	Autumn

Figure 7-3 Four Body Humors & Complemental Elements

Listed are the components of the Four Humors – blood, yellow bile, phlegm, and black bile, including element, temperature, moisture, personality, and season. If one looks closely, it is easy to see the interrelatedness of the categories. For example, phlegm is associated with cold and wet, and winter is the season when upper respiratory symptoms usually occur. Look again. Do you see any other "related" categories.

A lighter note referencing the humors was given by our tour guide in Annapolis, MD, *Squire Douglas,* who shared with us the four main ways to rebalance and restore health in the 18th and 19th century.

1. Since the **mouth** was the main entrance of the outside world into the body, an emetic was given to clean out the stomach
2. If you think the **stomach** was bad, you can imagine what is in the lower bowel. Therefore they gave cathartics.
3. Since **blood** carries disease through the body. Leeches and the scalpel were used to drain out the infirmities.
4. Lastly, **blistering** was used to drain infection out of the body. Redness and drainage caused by blistering the skin was evidence of the illness leaving the body. A hot coin was used.

Yin & Yang Theory

The above symbol, Yin (black) and Yang (white), represents the ancient Chinese understanding of the foundation of the universe. It is thought that the energies of yin and yang make everything happen. One element cannot exist without the other, they are complementary. Similar to hot and cold, Yin and Yang strives to balance contrasting elements. The Yin and Yang chart (Figure 7-4) shows the contrasts between them. If Yang, the masculine force, is overwhelming then there is excessive heat which injures the spirit. Severe pain follows.

Excessive cold, the feminine Yin factor, causes injury to the body creating swelling. Therefore, the onset of pain followed by swelling indicates that disharmony in the spirit has injured the body. But if swelling comes first, followed by pain, then disharmony in the body has harmed the spirit. Cure comes in the form of balance, mediating excessive heat or cold through the use of remedies such as herbal therapy, acupuncture, coining, or cupping.

In the case of the patient with an upper respiratory infection, symptoms may include cough, fatigue, and yellow sputum. A traditional healer may give a diagnosis of heat clogging the lungs, and prescribe acupuncture, herbal tea and rest in order to restore balance of Yin and Yang.

YIN	YANG
Female	Male
Cold	Hot
Darker	Lighter
Found inside body	Found on surface of body
Corresponds to night	Corresponds to day
Stands for confusion & turmoil	Stands for peace & harmony
Stands for conservation	Stands for destruction
Created earth	Created heaven

Figure 7-4   Yin & Yang Chart

Wind Theory

Once wind gets inside you, illness will occur. One day a Mexican American father brought his five year old daughter to the clinic. She had painful and frequent urination. From my biomedicine perspective and experience, I considered a urinary tract infection, vesicoureteral reflux, and possible sexual abuse, as a urinary tract infection symptoms are uncommon for children under the age of five. She looked well. I asked the father, "What do you think made her sick?" He responded, "When I took her outside the wind got inside of her."

The idea that wind, considered a menacing element, causes illness is a cultural health belief found in the Hmong, Cambodian, and Vietnamese cultures as well as Mexican. Symptoms congruent with the wind are fatigue, feeling of hot or cold, headache, restlessness, and decreased energy level. While these complaints could represent a variety of conditions, cure may come in the form of moxibustion (heat). It is a belief that heat has a therapeutic and balancing effect on the body, and through this process, wind is released and health restored.

Cures & other remedies

Coining is a heat treatment method frequently used to restore balance to the body. After an ointment is applied, a heated coin is placed on the affected site. The coin is pressed firmly against the skin and drawn down in one direction, hopefully without breaking the skin. This is repeated several times. If a dark blood appears under the skin, it is assumed that the treatment is working. If the site is only mildly red, the patient may need further treatments. On physical exam the HCP would see ecchymotic stripes in symmetrical rows. This would confirm that the patient did have "bad wind!"

Cupping, a similar method, is used when there is excessive Yin, as seen with sore muscles and body aches. A small heated cup-like form is applied to the skin, which causes a vacuum like suction to occur as it cools, thus rendering the noxious element ineffective and released from the body. Each application of a cup may take fifteen to twenty minutes. Again, on physical examination the HCP will see symmetrical, vertical rows of circular, non-raised, ecchymotic marks. It is thought that the greater the bruise, the greater the illness. This treatment is believed to remove cold elements and increase circulation.

Following the treatment, the patient is admonished to avoid taking a bath or drinking cold water because if water gets inside the body, it may block the wind from getting out, thus making symptoms worse. In talking with patients who hold a strong belief in this process, many will say they actually feel better after the treatment.

Restoring health may also come in the form of pinching. This procedure is especially effective with headaches, fatigue, loss of appetite, visual changes and to release wind from the body. For a headache, the procedure begins with rubbing a mentholated balm into the area, then placing the fingers and thumbs on both temples, slowing moving them in a massage like fashion across the forehead toward a spot between the eyes. The area between the eyes is then pinched and twisted. As with coining and cupping, if petechiae or ecchymosis occurs the treatment is deemed successful. It may be used on other areas of the body as well.

Massage provides yet another avenue to release the wind. Balm or lotion is rubbed onto the body to increase the blood flow, and to relax the muscles and the mind. Following the massage, the skin may be pinched and lifted to facilitate the release of the wind.

Other forms of Treatment

Acupuncture

The National Institute of Health has reviewed and scientifically analyzed several studies advocating the effectiveness of acupuncture. In 1997, a panel identified conditions that they felt would benefit from this adjunct therapy. These included addiction, stroke, rehabilitation, headache, carpal tunnel, and asthma.[10] In addition, the World Health Organization lists several conditions in which acupuncture is an effective treatment. These include upper respiratory infection, gastrointestinal issue, gynecological problems, and muscular disorders.

Acupuncture, a treatment based on Chinese medicine, has been around for thousands of years, but is just now recognized for its healing properties and only recently funded by some insurance companies. Considered a cold treatment to remove excessive Yang, it restores balance. The practice of puncturing the body to cure disease or relieve pain is done with a variety of needles, each having a specific purpose. Within the body, Chinese tradition asserts there is a vital life force called *Qi*. When the *Qi* is depleted or imbalanced, physical, emotional or mental illness can ensue. Meridians, the acupuncture sites for needle insertion, are thought to be the pathways where our *Qi* flows. Needle insertion rebalances this flow.

Sweat Lodge

On a visit to the Paiute Shoshone Indian Cultural Center in Bishop, California, our tour guide, a young Paiute Indian, shared information about his history and the cultural beliefs of his people. We discussed the sweat lodge and its healing properties. He must have gotten the sense that I needed healing because he offered to set up a time for a sweat lodge experience! I was surprised by his openness and generosity to someone not of native ancestry.

The Native American cultural belief of harmony and oneness with nature is revealed in the spiritual renewal and purification ceremony held in sweat lodges. Four recognized elements, fire, water, earth, and air are similar to those found in the Four Humors. These ceremonies, considered sacred events, can be used to heal an illness, to prepare for another ceremony or to seek guidance. Sage and sweet grass, both considered to have healing properties, are used along with cedar. Rocks are heated prior to the ceremony and placed in strategic locations. The doors are closed and prayers begin with a welcome for the spirits to join the participants.

Reiki

As HCPs, we cannot know every possible nontraditional treatment, but I am always amazed when I hear about a new form even though it has been around for hundreds of years. At a recent seminar I was presenting, a participant shared information about Reiki and now I'd like to share it with you. Reiki, was developed by Dr. Mikao in the 1880s in response to his students' inquiries about the healing abilities of Jesus and other spiritual healers. Reiki comes from two Japanese words, *rei,* which means "God's wisdom or higher power;" and *ki,* which is life force energy. It is the restorative nature that provides stress reduction and promotes healing. Placing one's hand just above the body and using various hand positions transfers the energy from the practitioner to the patient. Treating the whole person in this manner brings about feelings of peace, harmony and well-being.

Laughter Club

Laughter is the best medicine. The laughter club, first conceived by Dr. Madan Katana, a Bombay physician, takes advantage of the therapeutic value and contagious nature of laughing to promote wellness. There are over 400 clubs in India and 72% of the members report improved interpersonal relationships with co-workers, 85% say it has improved their self-confidence and 66% suggest that it has improved their ability to concentrate. We all need a little laughter every day!

Herbal Therapy

The decision when to pick herbs, where to pick, and how to prepare all determine the effectiveness of the therapy. At a recent Transcultural Nursing Society conference, I spent time with a Native Hawaiian registered nurse who was also a healer. As a child, she had been chosen by her grandfather to become the next healer in their community. She shared stories of leaving the house at midnight during a full moon in order to pick the herbs needed for her grandfather's patients. The tradition was passed from grandfather to granddaughter. Although she wants to write all this information down for the next generation, she has already met with resistance from her community as it is not in keeping with their oral tradition.

Herbs, like acupuncture, have become a part of mainstream medicine. While effective, they are not without possible side effects, thus discussion regarding their properties with patient's is essential. There are a multitude of herbs that have medicinal properties, and it is best to inquire if your patient is using them on a regular basis and for what purpose. Some of the commonly uses herbs are sage, chamomile, and ginseng.

Sage, used aromatically in the sweat lodge, is thought to purify and cleanse the body, mind and spirit. It may also be used for sleep, sore throat, breath cleansing and fever. It has been known to be used as a sage tea rubdown or bath as well as to drink or chew to cleanse the body's system of impurities. Chamomile, used by many as a means of relaxation, is thought to have a sedative and quieting effect, especially after a hectic day at work. Ginseng, a very popular herb, is thought to promote and improve male fertility as well as to enhance the immune system. For backpackers planning a trek at high elevations, it is said that taking Ginseng three days prior to a trip and then on the first two days on the trail, one can avoid altitude sickness. Since dehydration aggravates altitude sickness, it is vital to drink plenty of water at high elevations whether ginseng is used or not.

It is always best for the HCP to inquire about the herbs and over-the-counter treatments currently used by the patient and to discuss potential side effects and possible interactions with their current medications.

> *Reflective exercise ~ Healing treatments*
> 1. *What home remedies did your family use?*
> 2. *Were they helpful?*
> 3. *Do you still use them today?*
> 4. *Besides the healing treatments we discussed, what other healing modalities do your patients subscribe to in times of illness?*
> 5. *Are they incorporated into the plan of care?*

Healers

Healers have been the part of cultures for thousands of years. A Native American man at the Pomo Indian Conference shared that the elders of his tribe had selected him to be a healer. The young man was surprised by this, but then spent time in contemplation before responding to the request. In some cultures one may be "called" by the divine to serve as healer or identified by parents who deem their child ready to follow in their footsteps. This was the case of the Native Hawaiian registered nurse, whose grandfather selected her. Much of the information, beliefs, and practices are passed down from one generation to another orally. These cultural beliefs and health practices are considered believable and efficacious. Practices may include herbal therapy, massage, and a spiritual component as well, such as saying prayer, and lighting candles. Here is a list of healers from different cultural groups. Can you match them up?

> *Reflective exercise ~ Match the correct healer with their culture*
>
> | | | |
> |---|---|---|
> | 1. Curandero | | A. Korean |
> | 2. Folk Healer | | B. Roma |
> | 3. Kahuna | | C. Mexica |
> | 4. Hilot | | D. Hmong |
> | 5. Txiv Neb | | E. Euro American |
> | 6. Drabarni | | F. African Amer |
> | 7. Medicine man/woman | | G. Filipino |
> | 8. Physician/Nurse Practitioner | | H. Native American |
>
> *Answers*: 1-G: 2-F: 3-A: 4-G: 5-D: 6-B: 7-H: 8-E

Ancient wisdom, folk care practices, and healers are still an integral part of the lives of the patients we care for on a daily basis. Modern medicine is thought to have healing powers as well. The combination of the two modalities for some patients is the key to recovery from illness. Knowledge of your patient's cultural health practices leads to understanding and understanding to acceptance and respect. The goal is to provide quality care that integrates cultural beliefs and values into the plan of care. Culturally competent care is the result of both cultural awareness and knowledge. It is a journey. It begins anew every day. An inquisitive HCP seeks out information from the patient to assure that all possibilities have been uncovered. Together they develop a plan of care that incorporates cultural beliefs, values and health practices into the healing process.

Resources

Amerson, R. (2008). Reflections on a conversation with a curandera. *Journal of Transcultural Nursing.* (19)4, 384-387.

Andrews, M.M., Boyle, J.S. (2008). *Transcultural concepts in nursing care.* (5th Ed.). New York: Wolters Kluwer

Fadiman, A. (1997). *The Spirit Catches You and You Fall Down.* New York: Farrar, Straus and Giroux.

Foster, G.M. (1978). *Medical Anthropology* New York: John Wiley and Sons

Galanti, G.A. (2004). *Caring for patients from different cultures.* (4th Ed.). Philadelphia: University of Pennsylvania Press

Giger, J.N., Davidhizer, R.E. (2013). *Transcultural nursing: Assessment & intervention.* (6th Ed.). New York: Mosby.

Helsel, D., Mochel, M., Bauer, R. (2005). Chronic Illness and Hmong Shamans. *Journal of Transcultural Nursing.* (16)1, 150-154.

Hodge, F.S., Pasqua, B.A. Marquez, C.A., Cantrell, B.G. (2001). Utilizing storytelling to promote wellness in American Indian communities. J *Journal of Transcultural Nursing.* 13(1), 6-11.

Jackson, L.E. (1993). Understanding, eliciting, and genotiating patients' multicultural health beliefs. *Nurse Practitioner.* 18(4), 30-42.

Jones, P.S., Zhang, X.E., Siegl, K.J., Melies, A. (2002). Caregiving between two cultures: An integrative experience. *Journal of Transcultural Nursing.* (13)3, 210-217.

Leininger, MM.. (1991). *Culture care diversity and universality: A theory of nursing.* New York:National League for Nursing Press.

Leininger, MM.., McFarland, M.R. (2002). *Transcultural nursing: Concepts, theories, research and practice.* (3rd Ed.). New York: McGraw-Hill.

Lincoln, B. (2010). *Reflections from Common Ground: Cultural Awareness in Healthcare.* Wisconsin: PesiHealthcare

Lipson,J. G., Dibble, S.L., Minarik, P.A. (2001). *Culture & Nursing Care: A pocket guide.* San Francisco: UCSF Nursing Press

Marchione, M. (2009). Alternative medicine goes mainstream. *Napa Valley Register.*

McGoldrick, M., Giordano, J., Garcia-Preto, N. (2005). *Ethnicity and family therapy.* New York: The Guilford Press.

Purnell, L.D. (2013). *Transcultural health care: A culturally competent approach.* (4th Ed.). Philadelphia, PA: F.A. Davis Company

Sandoval, V.A., Adams, S.H. (2001). Subtle skills for building rapport using neuro-linguistic programming in the interview room. *FBI Law Enforcement Bulletin* 1-5.

Siatkowshi, A.A. (2007). Hispanic acculturation: A concept analysis. *Journal of Transcultural Nursing.* (18)4, 316-323.

Spector, R. (2012). *Cultural diversity in health and illness.* (8th Ed.), New Jersey: Pearson/Prentice Hall.

Thompson, S.B., Chien, E. (2006). Chinese medicine gaining respectability in west. *San Francisco Chronicle.* June 27, 2006.

Vigil, D. (2006). Thousands at cemetery for tomb sweeping rites. *San Francisco Chronicle.* April 3, 2006.

Vivian, C., Dundes, L. (2004). The crossroads of culture and health among the Roma (Gypsies). *Journal of Nursing Scholarship. (38)1,* 86-91

Yin and Yang. Retrieved October 2006 from www. Acupunture.com.au - Yin and Yang

Elsa's Story
Can you see me?

8

Emergency Preparedness & The Deaf Community

*A "failing grade" was given to the US Public warning
and emergency communication systems serving the
Deaf and Hard of Hearing post 9/11*

*Claude Stout - 2004
Emergency Preparedness and
Emergency Communication Access:
Lessons Learned Since 9/11 and Recommendations*

Unexpected. Unprepared. Uninformed. These are the some of the words people used to describe their disaster experience. Depending on where one lives in the United States, major disasters – earthquakes, tornados, hurricanes, snow storms and wild fires – have come their way. Vulnerable populations such as those with hearing loss, sight impairment, or limited ambulatory ability are at increased risk of injury and death during a disaster. There are warnings via sirens, TV/Radio and cell phone apps to alert the public. Now, imagine, in addition to being unprepared, you are deaf or hard of hearing (Deaf/HH). This adds another layer of anxiety and trepidation as you cannot hear the siren or radio alert.

Furthermore, hearing impaired persons, trapped inside a building, usually cannot hear emergency responders. Which begs the question – are emergency responders trained to meet the specific needs of the Deaf community in a disaster? In this chapter we address the needs of the hearing impaired and educational training for emergency responders and healthcare professionals

> *Reflective exercise: You've just experienced a disaster - earthquake, tornado, flood, hurricane . . .*
> 1. *What was your first concern?*
> 2. *What emotions surfaced?*
> 3. *Were you prepared? Did you have a plan? An emergency kit? Water & food for three days?*
> 4. *Now consider the same experience – from a Deaf person's perspective.*
> 5. *What additional items are essential during a disaster?*

Elsa's Story

Elsa is heading for the doctor's office on the Vine, the local bus. Her fractured wrist aches dully, but at least it's the left one. Crouching under the maple leaf table that night the shaking started was wise. If only she hadn't slammed her arm on the wall getting out of bed. Dr. Elmwood is pretty nice, thank heavens, for a hearing person. Elsa had met her the morning after the 7.0 temblor when she'd managed to get to the Queen of the Valley Hospital and see someone.

"*My bruises from the quake don't seem too big a deal any more, though my night alone at Embassy Suites in Napa is still really stark in my mind; something jostling me out of bed, the clock showing 3:20 AM, old film clips of elementary school drills Mrs. Potchatek showed us at Haman flashing before my eyes. I wish I'd come to this conference in the Valley with Francie, though. Sharing a room would have been cheaper, that's for sure. Another Deaf of Deaf friend would've made me feel more solid in the midst of the upheaval; she wouldn't have heard* the alarm either. And we could have calmed each other by quoting from <u>Never Seduce a Scot</u> or playing the Elephant Game."

The ASL interpreter was late, but is now there sitting beside the doctor in his office. Dr. Elmwood must have been on call in emergency when Elsa came in before. She tries to explain to this doctor how it's just a throbbing in her wrist now, but he keeps looking down at his notepad or at the screen with Elsa's medical history.

"Sure wish Dr. Elmwood was here, " Elsa muses. "She's always so focused on me. Maybe this guy thinks I can read his lips accurately! Fat chance."

Elsa gestures expansively with her good arm and leaps out of her chair as she tries to explain how the painkillers don't help at night. Dr. Stone steps back, startled. The quake itself was terrifying and disorienting, so that's probably part of the problem, but Elsa would really love something that would let her sleep for seven hours and wake up without feeling fogged in. Dr. Stone looks at the screen and mumbles to the interpreter about how the damage to Napa's buildings are so much more permanent than those to human "victims."

Defining Deaf

Deaf is defined three ways: Deaf, Culturally Deaf and deaf. Deaf, with a capital "D," refers to a culture, a community which holds the belief that deafness is not a disability, but rather a personality attribute. In the literal definition, *Deaf* persons in this category have profound hearing loss, use American Sign Language (ASL), and are acculturated into the Deaf community. Elsa considers herself a member of the Deaf community. *Culturally Deaf* are those who are deafened pre-linguistically, prior to age three. Deaf with a small "d" refers to persons who are partially deaf, hard of hearing.

They do not use ASL as their primary language, and are not considered acculturated into the Deaf community.[11] Hearing loss is defined as "a little trouble hearing," "moderate trouble," "a lot of trouble," or "deaf." They represent a distinct minority of less than one million persons living in the United States. The majority who have a hearing loss are age sixty and older.

Demographics

Being a Deaf/HH individual presents challenges to living in a hearing world. There are approximately ten million persons living in the United States who identify as Deaf. According the the 2012 Center for Disease Control Summary Health Statistics for U.S. Adults, 15% of those aged eighteen and older reported hearing trouble. The Gallaudet Research Institute (GRI) offered the following summary:[12]

Age	Population	Percent
> 6 years old	691,883	1.81%
Age 18-34	2,309,000	3.4%
Ages 34-44	2,380,000	6.3%
Ages 45-54	2,634,000	10.3%
Ages 55-64	3,275,000	15.4%
> 64 years	8,729,000	29.1%

Deaf individuals may have limited ability to read and comprehend information such as health education pamphlets. Almost 44% of Deaf students do not graduate from high school, and for those who do, only five percent graduate from college.[13] It is imperative for those who work in the healthcare or emergency services, to receive educational training and communication skills to ensure Deaf individuals receive culturally competent healthcare.

> *Reflective exercise: American with Disabilities Act 1990*
> 1. *Can you name all the disabilities covered by the original ADA?*
> 2. *The ADA expanded its definition in 2009 added what . . . and why?*
> 3. *Have you received training to care for the Deaf/HH patient?*
> 4. *Is your facility equipped to assist the Deaf/HH? The visually impaired? The non-ambulatory?*

History

The Americans with Disability Act of 1990 underlines the importance of equal access and equal care. Signed into law on July 26, 1990, by President George H.W. Bush, it was considered a civil right. It was patterned after the Civil Rights Act of 1964. The ADA, as it has come to be known, prohibits discrimination and ensures equal rights for housing, public accommodation, transportation, and employment. Additionally it provides opportunities to participate in state and local government programs and services. This act gave voice to the disabled, who prior to 1990, had not been considered a significant part of the population.

Disability, as defined by the ADA is *a physical or mental impairment that substantially limits one or more major life activities. This includes persons who have a history or record of such an impairment, or a person who is perceived by others as having such an impairment.* The initial definition of disability by the ADA in 1990 was so narrow that many persons did not qualify for services. As a result, people continued to face discrimination. In 2008 the Supreme Court ruled that the ADA was too narrowly defined, thus limiting access to resources for many disabled persons. In 2009 Congress passed the Americans with Disabilities Act Amendments Act (ADAAA) which broadened the definition of disability. The revised definition provided a broader scope of the term impairment and major life activities. While we are acquainted with the concept and purpose of the ADA, many of us are unaware of the specific disabilities covered in this amendment.

Impairment:

1. Any physiological disorder or condition, cosmetic disfigurement, or anatomical loss affecting one or more body systems, such as neurological, musculoskeletal, special sense organs, respiratory (including speech organs), cardiovascular, reproductive, digestive, genitourinary, immune, circulatory, hemic, lymphatic, skin, and endocrine; or

2. Any mental or psychological disorder, such as an intellectual disability (formerly termed "mental retardation"), organic brain syndrome, emotional or mental illness, and specific learning disabilities.

Major Life Activities: Major life activities include, but are not limited to:

- Caring for oneself, performing manual tasks, seeing, *hearing,* eating, sleeping, walking, standing, sitting, reaching, lifting, bending, speaking, breathing, learning, reading, concentrating, thinking, communicating, interacting with others, and working; and

- The operation of a major bodily function, including functions of the immune system, special sense organs and skin; normal cell growth; and digestive, genitourinary, bowel, bladder, neurological, brain, respiratory, circulatory, cardiovascular, endocrine, hemic, lymphatic, musculoskeletal, and reproductive functions. The operation of a major bodily function includes the operation of an individual organ within a body system.[14]

The definition was expanded to include the words "but not limited to," which ensures rights for the disabled. Furthermore, accreditation by The Joint Commission requires that the needs of Deaf/HH patients are met. Standards RI 2.1, 2.3 and 2.2 guarantee the rights of the patient to "adequate communication which includes the presence of professionals to provide translator/interpretive services." This include American Sign Language (ASL) translators. Furthermore, the Culturally Linguistically Appropriate Standards, developed by the Office of Minority Health, require all institutions to provide ASL interpreters, D/deaf telecommunication devices TTY/TDD; closed captioning television and real time video interpreting services. In addition, flashing light warning systems are required.

Barriers

National and international disasters often leave the Deaf/HH underserved. Why? One reason is that support organizations lack resources – staff time and the ability to create and distribute emergency preparedness material. In addition, emergency alerts, transmitted via television and radio, are not always accessible to the Deaf/HH community. Moreover, there is a wide variation in literacy rates. It is estimated that 30% of Deaf adults have weak ASL skills and can only read at a sixth grade level.[15] As a result, misunderstandings occur, especially in an emergency situations.

In addition to low literacy, Deaf/HH persons may be hesitant to seek health care because of their inability to communicate effectively or perhaps due to a bad experience with a HCP or clinic. As a consequence, the seeds of distrust may cause a reluctance to schedule future appointments. Likewise, as with many hearing patients, if the HCP is seen as paternalistic, condescending or demeaning, one's association with the health care system is affected. It is important to recognize the limitations of language and literacy and to provide services to meet their needs, thereby improving relationships and health outcomes.

Cultural Beliefs & Values

With the assistance of family, friends, educators and colleagues, Elsa has overcome obstacles in her life. However, when the earthquake struck, she was alone – without the support of her community. She had come to visit friends in the Napa Valley and was staying at a downtown hotel. While she was able to check in with ease, no mention of her special needs was noted on the reservation. As a result, desk personnel had no idea that she would not hear the alarm at 3:20 a.m. to evacuate the building.

Commitment and loyalty are the cornerstone of the Deaf community. As mentioned, they do not identify as disabled, but rather as a member of a distinct cultural group with a center on the linguistic. In the the book, *The People of the Eye,* the authors assert that deafness is an ethnicity and must be given its due, socially and politically. While Deaf identity is not based on religion, race or class "there is no more authentic expression of an ethnic group than its language."[16]

The Deaf culture, similar to other cultural groups, has a history, embraces values and beliefs, and use a specific language – ASL.

Cultural Beliefs & Values - Deaf Community

- Unity with other Deaf persons
- Use of American Sign Language
- Importance of Bilingual Education
- Communication - use of eye contact, gesturing & visual cues
- Music, films, literature, athletics, folklore that celebrate the Deaf culture

Communication

Stefany Anne Goldberg captures the essence of ASL language when she states that to properly ask a question you must "… first make a statement, then shrug your shoulders, cock you head to one side, open your eyes wide, and perhaps add an inquisitive expression to your face. To a hearing person this feels like overkill– like donning a Greek theater mask every time you need to find the bathroom. But communicating with your whole body is a fundamental part of ASL. It's a visual idiom, a language of the eye." [17]

American Sign Language is:

- A complete complex language
- Uses hands, facial gestures, and body posture to communicate
- Begins sentences with time, then noun, adjective & verb.
    - Physician says: You may need thyroid medication

- ASL interpreted as : In May, I'll need thyroid medication

- ASL may vary according to location, neighborhood, state and region

If a person became deaf pre-linguistically (usually before the age of three), they more likely use ASL as their form of communication. Other modalities that may be used in conjunction with ASL are Signed Exact English (SEE), Pidgin Signed English (PSE), Cued Speech, Lip Reading and the spoken word. Lip reading, long thought to be an effective method of communication, has proven less credible. Only 30-40% of spoken words are clearly understood. The sounds on the lips may look the same as other words, thus opening the door to misunderstanding.[18] Furthermore, for the Deaf, English is considered a "foreign language," therefore not understood easily. Similar to other languages, English words, especially medical terminology, do not exist in ASL. Health instructions, medication dosing, and warnings about adverse effects of medication are not easily translated. Potential misunderstanding may lead to poor health outcomes.

> *Reflective exercise: Communication/ Effective Ways to Communicate*
> 1. *List four risks to the Deaf patient when translation services are not available.*
> 2. *Do you sign? Are there ASL personnel available in your facility to translate?*
> 3. *What are some alternative methods you could use to convey a message to a Deaf patient?*

Family

The term *Deaf of Deaf* refers to Deaf parents who produce Deaf children. These children become acculturated into the Deaf culture and community. They use ASL as their primary language. Conversely, hearing children born to Deaf adults are known as *Children of Deaf Adults* (CODA). They generally use ASL as a primary language and learn English, their second language when they enter school. They are considered "culturally Deaf" because although they can hear, ASL is their first and primary language. Those who lose their hearing later in life are called "physically deaf" but "culturally hearing" because their primary language is the spoken word.[19]

In the past, parents did not know if their child was deaf until age three when it was expected that they "should be speaking." Today, screening programs designed to identify hearing loss in infants shortly after birth promotes early intervention and identification of resources for the parent and child. Regardless of a newborn's ability to hear, Deaf parents communicate with them using ASL, as it is their primary language. However, when a Deaf child is born into a hearing family this creates a challenge, especially if the parents use only the spoken language. In Elsa's case, her parents were "culturally hearing." Perhaps akin to Deaf parents who wanted their child to use ASL, her parents wanted her to learn English, as that was their primary language. Parents' perspectives and beliefs about hearing loss and communication may determine the direction that is taken. Early intervention, which includes discussion with experts and knowledge of options, allows parents to make an informed decision. Deaf parents of "hearing newborns" face the language decision. For Elsa's parents the benefit of early intervention was time – time to accept this diagnosis and to plan accordingly. A decision to learn ASL in combination with English, provided the communication skills that benefited her socially and academically. Likewise, her siblings learned a "new language" too. As she grew up, experiencing her family's love and support, she felt confident in her identity and purpose.

Health Care

From the Western medicine viewpoint, deafness is considered a pathophysiological condition in need of repair. Conversely, within the Deaf community, it serves as a proud identity and an appropriate descriptor for a deaf person. For those working in healthcare it is important to recognize the difference of opinion, and to acknowledge the pride held by those in the Deaf culture. This is the first step in establishing rapport and building a trusting relationship.

Healthcare institutions that insure that an ASL interpreter is available for the initial encounter demonstrate an understanding and acceptance of the patient's communication needs. Asking how one would like to be addressed and inquiring about family or support persons, prior to the discussion about the purpose of the visit, validates an interest in their well-being. During the appointment, it is imperative that the HCP listens attentively, acknowledge the concerns, and reflect a caring attitude. Usually, the visit closes when the HCP stands, closes the chart, and moves toward the door. However, in the Deaf culture these actions actually occur in reverse. Once the healthcare concerns have been addressed and resolved, the conversation (socialization) is expected to continue even as the patient prepares to leave. Important aspects of conversation to consider during a clinic/hospital conversation are:

- Acknowledge patient as a member of the Deaf community

- Create environment that promotes vision as primary sense

- Display consistent eye contact & visual attention

- Recognize visual signal/signs such as a pause, a facial expression to indicate essence of meaning of thought and/or conclusion to thought.

- Discern inclusion strategies such as waving, tapping shoulder, flicking light switch to get the persons' attention

- Insure interpreter is a certified translator versed in ASL and medical terminology. Interpreter should sit to the side or just behind the HC

Emergency Preparedness

The key to development and acceptance of Emergency Preparedness material for the Deaf community is collaboration with representatives from the Deaf/HH, EMT and HCP sectors. The educational material must include: cultural values and beliefs of the Deaf community, consideration of the educational level and literacy level of the person as well as examples of real-life scenarios. Determining quality and readability of written material is essential to assure clear understanding. The Department of Health and Human Services (DHHS) issued the *Quick Guide to Health Literacy* and its *Toolkit for Making Written Material Clean and Effective*. It provides the criteria for designing and evaluating educational pamphlets. The Suitability Assessment Method or SAM is an additional tool to insure that written material is clear and effective. An excellent example of such a pamphlet, *Disaster Preparedness and the Deaf Community*, was developed by the Red Cross in Rochester, New York in collaboration with members from the Deaf/HH community and Community Emergency Response Training (CERT) personnel. It is available online through the Rochester NY American Red Cross.

Cultural Awareness Education

A successful educational program for healthcare staff and emergency responders is contingent upon the belief that such a program is necessary and that participants have the desire to engage in the dialogue. In addition, the collaborative effort by members of the Deaf/HH, Emergency Responders and healthcare staff communities ensures attendance. An effective educational training program includes: an overview of the history of the ADA, the rights of the disabled, assessment of biases, barriers to care, cultural beliefs/values of the Deaf/HH, literacy level, communication and the identification of specific needs during a disaster. Presentation must include bilingual presenters – English speaking and ASL. Because the seminar material is developed by all parties, it gives credibility to the program. Outcomes include an assurance to the community that emergency responders and healthcare staff have the skills to care for the Deaf/HH in a disaster.

One such training is called the *Deaf Strong Hospital program*.[20] This educational training uses a role reversal to highlight the importance of interpreting services to improve cross-linguistic communication. Deaf volunteers serve as staff and HCPs. The hearing medical students are not allowed to speak and must act out illness scenarios. This training could be used for emergency preparedness programs as well. The hearing Emergency Responders and HCPs are disaster victims and the Deaf/HH are the first responders and health care staff. Each gain a heightened awareness and respect of needs of the other.

> *Reflective exercise: Health Education*
> 1. *What resources and support services are available in your community for the Deaf/HH?*
> 2. *Have you received inservice on caring for the Deaf/HH?*
> 3. *What health education material (pamphlets/videos) are available in your facility specifically for the Deaf/HH?*
> 4. *Do your support groups include signers?*

Conclusion

As HCPs and ERs, we may not be adequately prepared to care for Deaf/HH patients. Minimal experience, coupled with limited knowledge of the the Deaf culture leads to poor health outcomes. In order to provide quality competent care and advocate for the Deaf/HH, we must be knowledgeable about their rights, needs and our responsibilities.

HCP & ER Staff Caring for the Deaf/HH

Acknowledge & Affirm

Deaf is a Culture

Discuss & Adjust

Provide ASL Interpreters

Include Family

Collaborate and Change

Deafness is Not a Pathophysiological Condition

*   *   *

Press release on the 16th anniversary of the Americans with Disability Act

The promise of the ADA was that all Americans should have equal access and equal opportunity, including Americans with disability. The ADA was about independence and the freedom to make our lives what we will. We celebrate that today, and we recommit ourselves to ending discrimination in all its forms.

President Barak Obama, 2011

Resources

Altevogt, B.M., Pope, A.M., Hill, M.N., Shine, K.I. (2008). Research priorities in emergency preparedness and response for public health systems. Institute of Medicine. Washington, DC: The National Academies Press.

American Red Cross. (2005). Disaster preparedness and the Deaf community. Retrieved November 8, 2014 from www.RochesteRedCross.org

Andrade, P.C., de Carvalho Fortes, P., de Carvalho Fortes, P.A. (2010). Communication and information barriers to health assistance for Deaf patients. *American Annals of the Deaf.* 155:31-37.

Barnett, S. (2004). Cross-cultural communication with patients who use American Sign Language. *Family Medicine.* 34(5). pp. 376-382.

Blackwell DL, Lucas JW, Clarke TC. (2014). Summary health statistics for U.S. adults: National Health Interview Survey, 2012. National Center for Health Statistics. Vital Health Statistics. 10(260).

Chew, L.S., Bradley, K.A., Boyko, E.J. (2004). Brief questions to identify patients with inadequate health literacy. *Family Medicine.* 36(8). pp. 588-594.

Crowe, K., McLeod, S., McKinnon, D.H., Ching, T. (2012). Speech, sign, or multilingualism for children with hearing loss: Quantitative insights into caregivers' decision making. *Language, Speech and Hearing Services in Schools.* 45:234-247.

Engelman, A., Ivey, S.L., Tseng, W., Dahrouge, D., Brune, J., Neuhauser, L. (2013). Responding to the Deaf in disasters: Establishing the need for systematic training for state-level emergency management agencies and community organizations. *BMC Health Services Research.* 13:84-94.

Fileccia, J. (2011). Sensitive care for the Deaf: A cultural challenge. *Creative Nursing.* 17(4). pp. 174-179.

Galluadet Research Institute. (2014). About American Deaf Culture. www.gallaudet.edu

Glickman, N.S. (2009). Adapting best practices in CBT for Deaf and hearing person with language and learning challenges. *Journal of Psychotherapy Integration.* 19(4). pp. 354-384.

Goldberg, S. (2011). Can you see me now? Meet deaf American – a culture, a class, and a choice. *The Smart Set.* 5:14-15.

Harkins, J., Tucker, P.E., Williams, N., Sauro, J. (2010). Vibration signaling in mobile devices for emergency alerting: A study with Deaf evaluators. *Journal of Deaf Studies and Deaf Education.* 14(4). pp. 438-445.

Hoag, L., LaHousse, S.F., Nakaji, M.C., Sadler, G.R. (2010). Assessing deaf cultural competency of physicians and medical students. *Journal of Cancer Education.* 26:175-182.

Lane, H., Pillard, R.C., Helberg,U. (2011). *People of the Eye: Deaf Ethnicity and Ancestry.* New York: Oxford University Press

Macgregor-Skinner, G. Lim, A., Updike, A., Mazurek, A., (2014). Hearing-impaired patients require special consideration during a disaster. *Journal of Emergency Medical Services.* September. pp. 1-4.

Matthews, J.L., Parkhill, A.L., Schlehofer, D.A., Starr, M.J., Barnett, S. (2011). Role-reversal exercise with Deaf Strong Hospital to teach communication competency and cultural awareness. *American Journal of Pharmaceutical Education.* 75(3). pp. 1-10.

Neuhauser, L., Ivey, S.L., Huang, D, Engelman, A., Tseng, W., Dahrouge, D., Gurung, S., Kealey, M. (2013). Availability and readability of emergency preparedness materials for Deaf and hard-of-hearing and older adult population: Issues and assessments. *PLOS/ONE.* 8(2). pp. 55614-55625

Stout, C., Brick, K., Heppner, C.A. (2004). Emergency preparedness and emergency communication access: Lessons learned since 9/11 and recommendations. *Deaf and Hard of Hearing Consumer Advocacy Network.* pp. 1-40.

Sutton, V. (2013). Physical versus Cultural Deafness: Different languages mold different cultures. Retrieved November 3, 2014 from www.signwriting.org

U.S. Department of Labor. (2008). Accommodation and Compliance Series: The ADA Amendments Act of 2008. Office of Disability Employment policy. Retrieved November 3, 2014 from www.eeoc.gov/laws/statutes/adaaainfo.cfm

U.S. Census Bureau. (2013). Sex by age by hearing difficulty. 2013 American Community Survey. pp. 1-2. Retrieved November 3, 2014 from www.census.gov/factfinder/deaf

Jeremiah's Story...
Shut up & Listen

Urgent Care & Homeless Youth | 9

We've seen them – sitting in doorways, wandering the streets, talking to themselves, or standing at intersections with cardboard signs asking for donations. Homeless youth are a significant part of that landscape. They leave home for a variety of reasons – abuse (verbal, physical, sexual), unstable family relationships, drug usage, and mental illness. Living on the streets brings its own set of issues. Increased anxiety and stress often leads to poor decisions. They are at high risk for physical and sexual abuse. Low self-esteem and distrust of those in the healthcare system influence their decision whether to seek care. Life on the street usually equates to uncertainty and insecurity.

> *Reflective exercise: Homeless Experience*
> 1. *Have you or someone you know been homeless?*
> 2. *What image comes to mind of a homeless person? Homeless youth?*
> 3. *When you encounter a homeless person, do you interact with them, give them money or do you avoid eye contact?*
> 4. *If your teenage son or daughter were homeless, what would be your greatest fear?*

Jeremiah's Story

"Then he goes on about jumpin' the Q, and I lose it. I mean, just because I bumped into Mo in the food line don't mean I'm queer... So I had to rough him up a bit, ya know what I mean? Except that I didn't, really."

Jeremiah groans as he tries to stretch out his injured arm. The black fellow, who spoke with an odd accent and was pretty damn fit for someone waiting for soup, had really let go on him. Jeremiah's nose is still bloody, and his arm aches whenever he tries to scratch his armpit. He keeps forgetting. But every time he tries it hurts, almost as much as when his step-dad used to grab him for coming home later than 11PM. Wussy hour; 11! And Chuck was always loaded by then anyway. Amazing he even noticed that Jeremiah was late.

Sylvie listens attentively as Jeremiah goes on. Her step dad is an a-hole too, and she gets it. They share space under the overpass when it rains, besides. Jeremiah is righteous. Never even tried anything.

"Did you get any soup?" she asks. She cares about him, he knows. "I bet the clinic can help, J. Why don't you come down with me? I have an STD test this afternoon, and I bet the doctor will want to treat that arm."

"The last guy who saw me was a freak; kept asking about insurance and couldn't even get what I was saying. I mean, is 'coughing' such a hard word?? He was sure I was being taken by the DOJ, tied and headin' for "el carcel." Reminded me of Chuck. Why would I want to tell that guy anything? Let's go to Pull-a-Part instead, OK, Sylvie? They have good ops there for a quick five; all you gotta do is pound on some old clunker for a little lady who doesn't want to soil her britches---get her the bumper for her Buick Century wagon. Wanna come? I can check out the clinic later when I have a few bills."

Did you know?
- One in seven young people between the ages of 10 and 18 will run away
- Youth age 12 to 17 are more at risk of homelessness than adults
- 75% of runaways are female
- Between 20% and 40% of homeless youth identify as Gay, Lesbian, Bisexual, Transgender or Questioning (LGBTQ)
- 46 % of runaway and homeless youth reported being physically abused
  - 38% reported being emotionally abused
  - 17% reported being forced into unwanted sexual activity by a family or household member
- 75% of homeless or runaway youth have dropped out or will drop out of school

National Conference of State Legislatures (2010)[21]

What surprised you most about these statistics? Homeless youth, sometimes referred to as runaway youth, share a common background of neglect, family chaos, and a lack of structure in their lives. They are between the ages of fourteen and twenty four years of age. Many choose to live on the street or other transient shelter. They do not anticipate being homeless for a long period of time, but rather consider it a temporary adventure. Socialization with other homeless in the area assures economic survival.[22] The National Runaway Switchboard estimates that on any given night there are 1.3 million youth living unsupervised on the streets, in abandoned buildings, or residing with friends or strangers. Unfortunately, it is estimated that more than five thousand unaccompanied youth die each year as a result of assault, illness, or suicide.[23]

Barriers to care

Inadequate financial resources, lack of health insurance and transportation, are major reasons given for not seeking healthcare. In addition, anxiety about filling out forms, answering questions, and feeling self-conscious are also deterrents. They may have been told that health staff are required to contact their parents and/or social services because they are underage. It can be overwhelming to a young person who is already feeling uncertain and insecure to seek healthcare.

From the narrative we know that Jeremiah has had a negative experience with a healthcare provider, and is reluctant to make an appointment. From his (and homeless youth in general) perspective these are the major barriers.

Jeremiah's problems with HCP
- *Communicates disrespect*
- *Negative impression of health care received*
- *Perceived disinterest by staff*

Jeremiah wants HCP to
- *Recognize his personal health history & current issues*
- *Show respect for him*
- *Use nonjudgmental approach*

Homeless youth are three to four times more likely to die than the general population, and three to six times more likely to become ill due to poor access to healthy food and shelter. Perceived and real barriers promote a disconnect between them and the health provider. In addition, physical appearance and lack of social skills may lead to conflict and misunderstanding. Dissatisfaction with care may also lead to noncompliance resulting in hospitalization or death.[24]

Youth & Street Youth - Same Values - Find Common Ground

Youth Cultural Values & Beliefs
Autonomy
Testing of independence
Conformity with peer group
Preoccupation with clothes, hairstyles & grooming

There is diversity within this age group – roles and responsibilities, parental expectations, educational opportunities and economic options. Each play an integral role in the person's ability to face the challenges of growing up in today's society. Support and recognition of the transition from childhood to adolescence can vary from culture to culture. For example, Native Americans designate certain rites of passage for girls and boys as they grow into adulthood. In the Amish community, once the child has completed the 8th grade he/she leaves school and moves into a more significant role in the family structure.

Yet for many, adolescence is a time of experimentation. However, this is often seen by parents and medical staff as a time of risk taking behavior coupled with poor judgement. There is some physiologic truth to parents/HCP's view. The adolescent brain is still developing, consequently, decisions may not be well thought out. From Erikson's psychosocial development theory, adolescence is a time of Identity versus Confusion – asking the question "Who am I?" It is during this stage that a twelve to eighteen year old develops a sense of self and forms a personal identity. This exploration takes precedence in their life, and as a result these feelings of insecurity, it leads to conflict with parents, teachers and authority figures. Continual acrimony with parents, and one's peer group, can influence the decision to runaway.

A home environment filled with physical and/or emotional abuse can be the impetus to leave. The "family" on the street may provide an opportunity for personal autonomy, and a connectedness that seems missing from their lives. What attracts them to venture from home into a world of uncertainty? Street culture offers them:

Street Youth Cultural Values & Beliefs

Sense of value and connectedness

Personal autonomy

Reliance on peers

Interdependence

Shared mistrust of authority figures

Reflective exercise: Cultural Beliefs/Values
1. *Describe the similarities of youth and street culture youth.*
2. *What is the biggest challenge to providing care to the homeless youth?*
3. *List ways you'd try to establish a respectful and trusting relationship.*
4. *How does your healthcare facility reach out to homeless youth?*

Communication . . . "Shut up and listen"

That was the response given by a young person in a focus group when asked the **question** – W*hat can healthcare providers do to help homeless youth feel that they care about the issue being discussed?* **Answer** . . ."Shut up and listen!"[25] Unfortunately, street youth perceive the HCP as disrespectful and lacking in empathy. From the HCP's viewpoint, street youth appear disinterested, vague and distant.

Jeremiah, and many youth like him, experience a sense of powerlessness with those in authority. As a result they avoid encounters. To compensate for this they may appear more aggressive in their mannerism. The remark of one young homeless woman summarizes the concept well – "I think that, if I was ever to go to a counselor again I would actually want them to like hear me out and understand me, what I'm saying to them about my life and how I am feeling . . . ."[26]

The youth's style of communication usually reflects the unique jargon of their peer group. Their response to a question can vary from a blank stare, a one word answer or long periods of silence. Moreover, the tone of the conversation may be determined by the events of the day for both the youth and the HCP. If already stressed due to an overbooked schedule, the HCP may appear disinterested or tired. Financial concerns or lack of insurance may increase the anxiety of the young person. As a result, the success of the encounter is affected by both. In addition, a reluctance to talk about sensitive issues or concerns about confidentiality, can create a barrier to gathering vital health information. As the HCP actively listens and demonstrates a genuine interest in the youth's concerns, opportunities to gain their confidence, respect, and trust are possible. Beginning the conversation with "yes" or "no" questions, and then progressing to open-ended questions is an effective technique.

Fully engaged conversations by both parties offers the a moment to acknowledge differences and establish rapport. Building a trustful adolescent-HCP relationship is the cornerstone to a successful outcome. It is important to refrain from using medical jargon. As you examine the patient, share your findings. Share with the patient what is considered normal and what is not. Once a diagnosis is made, engage them in the conversation.. What are their concerns and suggestions?

> *Reflective exercise: Communication ~ Getting to the heart of the message?*
> 1. *Did the phrase "shut up and listen" surprise you?*
> 2. *How do you establish rapport with youth?*
> 3. *What communication techniques do you use to 'listen more?'*
> 4. *What if the patient continues to give 'one word' answers or not respond – how would you to change your approach?*

Health Care Options . . . What works – What doesn't!

Locus of control for many youth may be externally motivated. Given that at their age cognitive functioning is more concrete, many chose to manage their health with self-care treatments. If unresolved, they often seek the advice of their peer group. Making an appointment at a health clinic may be last on their list of options. Concerns about confidentiality, especially when identification is required, may deter the call. So what can we as HCPs do to create an environment that welcomes homeless teenagers as well as provides a safe haven for open discussions and collaborative care?

Homeless youth are more likely to respond affirmatively and to engage in collaborative dialogue when the clinic staff emanates understanding and sensitivity for their issues. A welcoming environment occurs when the needs and culture of the youth are acknowledged. Peer groups, especially for the homeless youth, are vital to the sense of well-being and security. Therefore, encouraging friends to accompany the youth into the exam room promotes a sense of safety and security. Additionally, drop-in centers are viewed as flexible, accessible and offer a link in the network of support. They also can promote available resources.

Keys to Care

Encouraging peers to accompany the patient to the exam may be the most positive step in the process. In our narrative, Sylvie encourages Jeremiah to come with her to the clinic. Once there, she may encourage him to make a same day appointment, letting him know that she would accompany him. This provides Jeremiah with confidence to address his current issue. Sylvie can add important information to the conversation as well. This three-way dialogue is an opportunity to identify concerns not previously mentioned. When the HCP demonstrates a genuine interest and displays a non judgmental attitude, barriers are eliminated and quality care is given.

From this encounter the word gets out to the homeless in the youth community that this is the place to go for all services – health, referrals, counseling, and preventative care. Listed are the qualities youth want from mental healthcare providers.

Keys to Caring for Homeless Youth

- Be nonjudgmental
- Have a good sense of humor
- Empower rather than enable
- Offer choices instead of advice
- Build trust by being honest regarding confidentiality and the limits of confidentiality
- Be patient and not give up on them

- Match the treatment with the youth instead of matching the youth with the treatment
- Be aware of their own personal problems[27]

> *Reflective exercise: Keys to providing quality care to youth*
> 1. *Take a moment to consider each point.*
> 2. *Which reflects your style and attitude?*
> 3. *Is is always effective?*
> 4. *Is there anything you'd add to the list?*
> 5. *What other techniques have you tried?*

Taking it to the Streets

How can we reach out to homeless youth to inform them of our services. In an article called *Postcards from the Edge: Collaborating with young homeless people to develop targeted mental health messages and translate research into practice*, researchers collaborated with homeless youth to develop effective health messages which included practical information about mental health services and managing medications for homeless youth.[28] The youth were asked to come up with images and quotes that they felt reflected a young homeless persons experience. In all they produced a series of ten postcards. The focus of these postcards was to disseminate information about mental health and medication. However, this could be expanded to include health promotion, preventative care, vaccinations, immunizations and sex education.

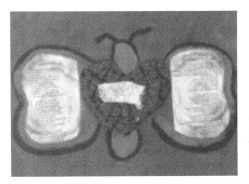
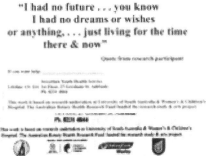

Figure 9-1 Postcards From the Edge

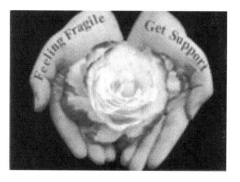 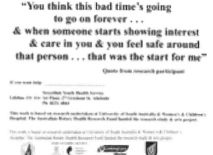

Figure 9-2 Postcards From the Edge

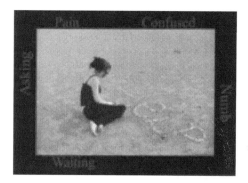 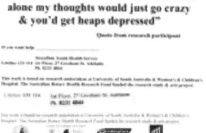

Figure 9-3 Postcards From the Edge

Muir-Cochrane, E., Oster, C., Drummond, A., Fereday, J., Darbyshire, P. (2010). 'Postcards from the Edge': Collaborating with young homeless people to develop targeted mental health messages and translate research into practice. *Advances in Mental Health.* Used with permission.

Summary

There are a multitude of ways that we can reach homeless youth. Key elements are creating a welcoming environment, encouraging open and engaging conversations, and acknowledging the importance of peer support. Creating a safe place to share their health concerns – mental, physical and emotional – sends a message of genuine interest in their well-being. As a result they are more likely to return for follow up care and treatment. Each encounter is an opportunity for homeless youth to connect with educators, counselors and housing coordinators. It is this collaborative effort that gives rise to successful and healthy outcomes.

A Collaborative Approach to Ensure
Positive Health Outcomes & Trusting Relationships

Acknowledge & Affirm
Promote Autonomy
Ensure Confidentiality
Acknowledge importance of peer support

Discuss & Adjust
Encourage Peer Involvement
Nutritional concerns & resources
Communication with family

Collaborate & Change
Unhealthy behavior
Substance abuse
High risk concerns

Resources

Barry, P.J., Esign, J., Lippek, S.H. (2002). Embracing street culture: Fitting health care into the lives of street youth. *Journal of Transcultural Nursing.* 13(2). p145-152.

Bunsen, N.H., Engebretson, J.C. (2008). Facilitating risk reduction among homes and street-involved youth. *Journal of the American Academy of Nurse Practitioners.* 20: 567-575.

Conn, M.A., Marks, A.K. (2014). Ethnic/Racial differences in peer and parent influence on adolescent prescription drug misuse. *Journal of Developmental & behavioral Pediatrics.* 35(4). pp. 257-265.

Desantis, L., (2001). Health-culture reorientation of Registered Nurse students. *Journal of Transcultural Nursing.* 12(4). pp. 310-318.

Ensign, J., Panke, E. (2002). Barriers and bridges to care: Voices of homeless female adolescent youth in Seattle, Washington, USA. (2002). *Journal of Advanced Nursing.* 37(2). pp. 166-172.

Ensign, J., Panke, E. (2002). Young homeless women encountered physical and individual barriers in obtaining health care. *Evidence-Based Nursing.* 5(14). pp.124-128.

Hardoff, D., Schonnmann, S. (2001). Training physicians in communication skills with adolescents using teenage actors as simulated patients. *Medical Education.* 35:206-210.

Hollywood Homeless Youth Partnership. (2010). A practical guide for service providers: Addressing intimate partner abuse in runaway and homeless youth. pp.1-27.

Hudson, A.L., Nyamathi, A., Sweat, J. (2008). Homeless youths' interpersonal perspectives of health care providers. *Issues in Mental Health Nursing.* 29:1277-1289.

Hunt, R.J., Swiggum, P. (2007). Being in another world: Transcultural student experiences using service learning with families who are homeless. *Journal of Transcultural Nursing.* 18(2). pp. 167-174.

Muir-Cochrane, E., Oster, C., Drummond, A., Fereday, J., Darbyshire, P. (2010). 'Postcards from the Edge': Collaborating with young homeless people to develop targeted mental health messages and translate research into practice. *Advances in Mental Health.* 9(2). pp. 138-147.

National Alliance to End Homelessness. (2006). Homelessness in the United States of America. Washington DC: National Alliance to End Homeless

National Council of State Legislatures. (2010). Homeless and runaway youth. Retrieved July14. 2014 www.ncsi.org/issues-research/human-services/homeless-and-runaway-yout.aspx

Witte, P. et al. (2012). The State of Homelessness. Washington DC: National Alliance to End Homelessness. Retrieved July 15, 2014 from www.endhomelessness.org

Rabinowitz, S., Schneir, A., Clark, L. (2010). No way home: Understanding the needs and experience of Homeless youth in Hollywood. Hollywood Homeless Youth Partnership. pp. 1-66.

Rew, L., Whittaker, T.A., Taylor-Seehafer, M.A., Smith, L.R. (2005). Sexual health risk and protective resources in gay, lesbian, bisexual, and heterosexual homeless youth. *Journal for Specialist in Pediatric Nursing.* 10(1). pp. 11-19.

Rundio, A.R. (2013). Health policy watch: Adolescent addictions. *Journal of Addictions.* 24(3). pp. 201-202.

Schneir, A., Stefanidis, N., Mounier, C., Ballin, D., Gailey, D., Carmichael, H., Battle, T. (2007). Trauma among homeless youth. *National Child Traumatic Stress Network.* Retrieved July 16, 2014 from www. NCTSN.org

Slesnick, N., Kang, M.J., Bonomi, A.E., Prestopnik, J.L. (2008). Six and twelve-month outcomes among homeless youth accessing therapy and case management services through an urban drop-in center. *Health Services Research.* 43(1). pp. 211-229.

U.S. Department of Health and Human Services. (2009). Psychological first aid for youth experience homelessness. National Child Traumatic Stress Network. pp.1-12. Retrieved July 15, 2014 from www. NCTSN.org.

Ev's Story

I'm not going back . . . | 10

Cancer - Lesbian Community

    The screen door to Mountolive Holistic slams, but doesn't quite close. Ev hardly notices as she enters. She has just come from Dr. Lenhardt's office and "the diagnosis." She hasn't even been home to tell Amanda yet. Thanks heaven that here, with Kara and her associates, she is treated with respect, even though she wonders whether their needles will have any effect at all on her cervix. Cancer. What a dreadful word.
    "A joint will make this better," she whispers. "Probably not needles."
    Ev and Amanda have been together for twenty years. Amanda's mom and stepdad live across the country in Rhode island and treat the couple as if they are roommates. Ev plays softball for the Rincon Valley Renegades and Amanda always wears skirts even though she spends her weekdays jumping around with a bunch of preschoolers, but the Riordans never speak of the two as a couple. They are roommates. Ev's family has disowned her altogether. If only she and Amanda

had been able to afford insurance without groveling. Mercy Clinic wouldn't recognize them as a couple, but Ev's parents certainly could have helped with some cash.

Herman Lenhardt, the Ob-Gyn Ev had found online, has offices near enough to their home on Oak Street so that no long bus trip was required. He'd been pretty brusque with the pap smear last week and seemed about as interested in Ev's relationship with Amanda as the Riordans. Don't ask. Don't tell. If he'd thought it odd that Amanda had wanted to be in the room during the exam, he hadn't said so. She was rather pretty really, unlike his fat patient. Dr. Lenhardt must have sensed that Ev's last doctor had been even rougher than he was and equally uncomfortable with forceful women. She did seem pretty vulnerable lying open-legged on the table in any case

This is a true story, one of many that I've heard. This narrative is reflective of others in the Lesbian Gay Bisexual Transgender (LGBT) community who have faced similar circumstances and challenges within the healthcare setting. Fears surrounding disclosure raises anxiety, thus hesitancy to seek care results. Uncertain of the response and treatment by the HCP, many lesbians forego an annual female exam and pap smear. Ev knew something was wrong. However, based on her previous negative experience with pelvic exams and rough handling by physicians, she chose to delay scheduling an appointment that perhaps could save her life. Yet when faced with discrimination on multiple levels, her once treatable disease is now terminal.

In addition to disclosure and discrimination, economic barriers determine access to healthcare. Lesbians are less likely to have adequate health insurance and are more likely to be uninsured. Consequently, scheduling recommended screenings is infrequent. As a result there are increased rates of breast and cervical cancer in lesbians. Perhaps if the clinic created a welcoming environment, and staff had received sensitivity training to care for LBGT patients, Ev would have entered the system earlier.

> *Reflective exercise: Comfort level . . .*
> 1. *Have you ever been in a medical office that made you so uncomfortable that you wanted to walk out?*
> 2. *Did you walk out?*
> 3. *If so, did you inform the HCP and staff of the reason for that decision?*
> 4. *If not, Why not?*
> 5. *Today, if in a similar situation, would you handle it differently?*

History . . . from then until now

On April 27, 1953 President Eisenhower invoked Executive Order 10450, Security Requirement for Government Employment. It legitimized dismissal if a government employee displayed "Any criminal, infamous, dishonest, immoral, or notoriously disgraceful conduct, habitual use of intoxicants to excess, drug addiction, sexual perversion." More than 1,000 people lost their jobs. In the era of McCarthyism, disclosure of being homosexual was equated to being a spy for a communist country. Federal and state mandates made the fear of losing one's teaching credential, custody of their children or dismissal from a government position a real possibility. Additionally, homosexuality was considered a mental disorder by the American Psychiatric Association (APA). It was listed in the Diagnostic and Statistical Manual of Mental Disorder (DSMA). Electroshock therapy was the treatment du jour. It was not until 1973 that the APA removed it from the DSMA.

Isolation and discrimination were commonplace. Change came in the late 1960's with an incident that took place at the Stonewall Bar which served people in the Gay community of New York City. After years of harassment and routine raids by the police, the patrons decided they "weren't going to take it anymore." Three days of rioting ensued. This was the beginning of The Gay Rights Movement – a campaign for civil and equal rights.

Unfortunately it took decades until institutions responded to this injustice with words and actions. In 1990 the World Health Organization removed it from its list of diseases. The 1993 "Don't ask, don't tell" law that allowed gays to serve in the military as long as they kept their sexual orientation private, was repealed in 2010. The seminal event that changed the lives of millions in the LGBT community was the ruling by the Supreme Court on June 26, 2013. It decreed that supporters of Proposition 8, the California law recognizing marriage as between a man and a woman, had no legal right ("standing") to appeal to the previous federal court's decision. Furthermore, the court struck down Section 3 of the Defense of Marriage Act (DOMA) which required the Federal government to treat same sex couples as unmarried. As a result, the Federal government was prohibited from granting Federal benefits, protection and responsibilities based on marriage. This seminal event was the stepping stone on the journey to equality.

Demographics & Definitions

As previously stated demographics "are only as good as the people who fill out the forms." Yet, what if the form did not provide a section to identify a specific group? Does that mean they did not exist? Are biases getting in the way of gathering pertinent data from which insights can be gained?

Depending on the source, it is estimated that between 4-10% of U.S. adults identify as LGB and 0.2 - 0.4% as transgender. This equates to over 9 million people. Discrepancies in data may be due to the "invisibility" factor in which persons choose not to self-identify. However, data gathering is changing. The 2000 Census allowed gay/lesbian couples to self-identify by asking the question of their sex and relationship to the "main householder."

Terms & Acronyms:

- *Bisexual* ~ a person whose sexual & romantic attraction is to both sexes
- Gender Identity ~ a person's sense of being a woman, a man or gender neutral.
- *Gay* ~ an attraction and/or behavior which focuses on someone from the same sex or gender identity
- *Heterosexual* ~ persons whose sexual and romantic attraction is the opposite sex or gender identity.
- *Lesbian* ~ refers to female same sex attraction and sexual behavior*

- *Queer* ~ a term that previously had been considered derisive and has been reintroduced as an umbrella term to identify gay, lesbian, transgender, bisexual, or any sexual anatomy or gender identity.
- *Questioning* ~ one's gender, sexual identity, sexual orientation
- *Partner* ~ a person's significant other exclusive of gender.
- *Sexual orientation* ~ referring to a person's physical and/or emotional attraction to the same and/or opposite sex.
- *Transgender* ~ a person whose birth identification differs from self gender identification or gender expression
- *Transexual* ~ a medical term that applies to those seeking medical/surgical treatment to live as a member of a sex category that is different than birth sex identification.
- LGBT has expanded to LGBTQ with Q referring to either queer or questioning.

Health Disparities

Negative experiences with healthcare providers, lack of insurance, and low socioeconomic status are reasons why many lesbians do not schedule preventative healthcare and screenings. Health disparities result. Lesbians have five times the risk for anxiety disorder and depression, and are more likely to attempt suicide than their heterosexuals.[29] Why? Bjorkman suggests that it is related to the effects of marginalization which lead to anxiety, depression, increased alcohol consumption, substance abuse and suicide.[30] Healthy People 2020 proposes that disparities are due to social stigmatization, discrimination, and the denial of civil and human rights. As a result some of the most pervasive health related issues faced by lesbians are:

- Alcoholism
- Substance abuse
- Depression/Anxiety/Suicidal ideation
- Smoking (2X more likely than general public)
- Obesity
- Cancers (cervical & breast)[31]

The Institute of Medicine Report *The Health of Lesbian, Gay, Bisexual & Transgender People* disclosed that research is not conducted evenly across sexual and gender minorities. They encourage researchers to develop innovative ways to conduct research, specifically with small populations such as the LGBT community. In addition, other factors that need consideration are the overlap between identity, behavior and desire (may engage in same sex behavior but do not identify as LGBT), the lack of research about the specific health needs of the LGBT population, and a reluctance of individuals to answer survey question about stigmatized identity and behavior.

In 2010 President Obama requested then Secretary of Health and Human Services (HHS) Kathleen Sebelius, to identify steps that the department could take to improve the health and well-being of LGBT individuals, families, and communities. In 2011 recommendations were sent to the President. and made public. The report recommended the inclusion of sexual orientation questions on the National Health Interview survey, and that all HHS programs establish sexual orientation and gender identification non discrimination policies.

Responding to the Call for Equality

•2004 American Psychological Association resolution
"Opposes any discrimination based on sexual orientation in matters of adoption, child custody and visitation, foster care and reproductive health services.

•2005 AMA Policy on LGBT Issues
H-65.990 Civil Rights Restoration. The AMA reaffirms its long-standing policy that there is no basis for the denial to any human being of equal rights, privileges, and responsibilities commensurate with his or her individual capabilities and ethical character because of an individual's sex, sexual orientation, gender, gender identity, or transgender status, race, religion, disability, ethnic origin, national origin, or age.

•2008 American Association of Colleges of Nursing
Provide resources to improve culture competence including those related to the health needs of LGBT.

• 2009 The Joint Commission Standard# R1.0101.01
Allows the presence of a support individual of the patient's choice and that the hospital adopt policies barring discrimination based on factors including sexual orientation and gender identity or expression.

•2010 Section 1557 of the Affordable Care Act
Provides for federal nondiscrimination protection in the health care system, including on the basis of "sex." The Office for Civil Rights clarified that this prohibition includes discrimination based on gender identity and sex stereotyping.

• 2012 The Joint Commission added
Advance effective communication and cultural competence in patient and family centered care for the LGBT community.

•2014 Healthcare Bill of Rights - LGBT HealthLink
- Right to be treated with equality and respect
- Right to affirmation of your true gender identity
- Right to help designating who will make decision for you
- Right to visitation by anyone you choose
- Right to your privacy
- Right to protections if you are discharged due to discrimination

> *Reflective exercise: Standards & Polices*
> 1. *Does your institution have policies that reflect these standards?*
> 2. *Has staff received inservice on the standards and application for accreditation?*
> 3. *From your perspective, are employees aware of the policies? Do they implement?*
> 4. *Is there more that can be done to increase awareness?*

The HCP's comfort level addressing sexual identity can influence decisions about care and treatment options. Assuming everyone is heterosexual, or that one's sexual orientation is not relevant can lead to poor health outcomes. We do know that lesbians have lower rates of recommended screening, thus are at increased risk for cervical and breast cancer. Skirting the discussion is not an option.

Now that we know . . . Some questions to ask ourselves
- Do we assume heterosexuality for every patient?
- Do we inquire about sexual orientation?
- Do our forms provide options for self-identification?
- How do our patients wants to be identified? What pronoun to use?
- How do they want their partner addressed?

Routinely asking about sexual orientation with all patients increases one's comfort level with the conversation. Unfortunately though, when someone shares their identity, an assumption of exactly what that means may be misinterpreted. Asking the patient to "tell me more about what that identity means to you" ensures the clarity needed to address potential and real health issues. Let's look at the following two scenarios.

Two Scenarios – Two Approaches . . . You Chose

Scenario 1:
You enter the waiting room of the OB/GYN clinic and walk to the receptionist. She does not make eye contact as she asks you about your health coverage and confirms your place of residence. Once the information is collected she asks you

to have a seat. You sit down. You feel uneasy as you look around. The pictures on the walls depict heterosexual couples with their children and white women at different life stages of life. The images on their educational pamphlets do not resemble you. You're ready to walk out when the receptionist calls your name and says "Mrs Smith the doctor will see you now." You're not married!

> *In the waiting room in your clinic or hospital . . .*
> 1. *Do the pictures on the walls reflect same sex couples? Heterosexual couples? With children?*
> 2. *Do the health brochures reflect the diversity of the community served?*
> 3. *Does the registration form include section for gender identity?*
> 4. *Have staff attended LGBT patient care educational seminars?*

Scenario 2:
You enter the waiting room of the OB/GYN clinic and walk to the receptionist. She greets you with a cheery hello and welcomes you. As this is your first visit to the clinic, the receptionist, in addition to asking about your health insurance status, and asks how you would like to be addressed. Wow, that was unexpected! As you sit down you notice the diversity of pictures on the walls depicting various ethnic groups, heterosexual and same sex couples with children. You are starting to feel more comfortable. As you reach down to pick up a periodical you realize that great care has been taken to meet the diverse needs of the clinic's population. Now, you're glad you came as they call your name "Janet, the doctor will see you now."

Strategy 1 – Creating a Welcoming Environment

It seems minor, but in reality, creating a waiting room that welcomes everyone with respect and dignity may make the difference in discovering cervical cancer, diagnosing vaginosis, or detecting a breast lump. Beginning with the receptionist greeting and inquiring how one would one like to be addressed to the diversity of photos displayed and the non-discrimination policy posted for all to see provides additional assurance. Moreover, the placement of educational brochures on LGBT health topics demonstrates an awareness of the health needs of women.

Ideally, a patient enters the waiting room, is greeted by the receptionist, called by name by the medical assistant and welcomed into the practice by the HCP. Every aspect is essential when establishing this new relationship. The HCP could begin by asking the patient to "tell me something about yourself." Taking an open and non-judgmental social and sexual history is key to building rapport. Here are some additional questions to ask. Are you in a relationship? What do you call your partner? Do you have any concerns about your sexuality, sexual orientation or sexual desires? What pronoun do you use to describe yourself?

The Institute of Medicine suggests the inclusion of structured data fields on the intake form to obtain information on sexual orientation and gender identify. Here is a example of data information suggested by the Fenway Institute.[32]

Do you think of yourself as:
    __ Lesbian/gay, or homosexual
    __ Straight or heterosexual
    __ Bisexual
    __ Something else_____
    __ Don't know

Strategy 2 - Improving Provider Knowledge

Education and training of staff is the cornerstone to providing quality care that meets your LGBT patients' needs. Staff who have received diversity training are more likely to extend hospitality and exhibit professionalism. Educational seminars need to include a review of history, health disparities, barriers to care, health risk factors specific to the LGBT patient. Integrating self-reflective and group exercises offers the participants insights into their beliefs and biases regarding the LBGT patient. s.

In addition, providing opportunities to practice gender neutral communication and ask sexually sensitive questions increases the comfort level of health staff to pursue that inquiry. Sensitive questions are always the most challenging. Yet, phrasing them in a way that connotes genuine interest invites responses. Here are some of the questions I ask my patients."How do you describe your sexual orientation and behavior?" Another possible question, "Do you have any concerns about your sexuality, sexual orientation or sexual desires? I usually preface these questions with the statement "I ask all my patients these questions." It is important that they know you are inclusive and follow a protocol to ensure that your are giving the best care.

Preventative Care & Screening

Recognizing the increased health risk for depression, anxiety, alcohol abuse, smoking and domestic abuse, the following screening tools may be helpful to obtain further information.

1. Alcohol Usage: CAGE Questionnaire screening
2. Depression: Beck's Depression Inventory
3. Smoking
4. Spirituality: Faith Assessment
5. Domestic abuse

In addition to the above screening tools, this is a great opportunity to discuss the relationship between infrequent screenings and risk of cancer. The current recommendation of the U.S Preventative Health Services is for **all women** to have a pap smear, which includes screening for the human papilloma virus (HPV), beginning at age 21; then every three years until age 29, and every five years thereafter until age 65. Lesbian and bisexual women are just as likely as heterosexual women to develop cervical cancer. Unfortunately they are ten times less likely to undergo regular screening. One study found HPV in almost 30% of women who only had sex with women.[33] As a result information regarding HPV transmission – skin to skin, oral to vaginal, digital vaginal genital contact – is vital for patients to know. It is important to inform them that infectious pathogens, such as Chlamydia, and Trichomoniasis, are shed in vaginal secretions and can lead to infection as well. The more information the patient has about this topic, the more likely she'll make healthy decisions about screening and care.

> *Reflective exercise: Asking the question & Being informed*
> 1. *Which of the screenings are the most comfortable to ask about?*
> 2. *Which ones are most difficult?*
> 3. *Prior to reading this section, were you aware of the modes of transmission for HPV or vaginal infections?*
> 4. *How could you share this information effectively with your patients using non-medical terminology?*

Summary

Our goal is to create a welcoming environment that embraces diversity. It is within this environment that we ensure that our lesbian patients receive preventative screenings and information specific to their health issues. It is essential that health staff address their potential biases, receive sensitivity training and education about the specific health needs of the lesbian patient. Sensitive and competent health care follow.

Recommendations for Health Care Providers[34]

Awareness & Asking the Right Questions

."How do you describe your sexual orientation and behavior?"
"Do you have any concerns about your sexuality, sexual orientation or sexual desires?
What pronoun would you use to describe yourself?

Attitudes Toward Homosexuality

Recognize and acknowledge beliefs and bias toward lesbian orientation

Medical knowledge & Screening for Specific Health Concerns of the Lesbian Patient

Safe sex
Transmission of disease between women
Anxiety/depression
Alcohol abuse
Domestic violence

Resources

Abdessamad, H.M., Ydin, M.H., Tarasoff, L.A., Radford, K.D., Ross, L.E. (2013). Attitudes and knowledge among Obstetrician-Gynecologist regarding Lesbian patients and their health. *Journal of Women's Health.* 22(1). 85-93.

Ard, K.L., Makadon, H.J. (2014). Improving the health care of lesbian, gay, bisexual and transgender (LGBT) people: Understanding and eliminating health disparities. *The Fenway Institute.* Retrieved September 14, 2014 from www.thefenwayinstitute.org

Bernstein, C. (2012). Addressing the needs of LGBT people in community health centers: What the governing board needs to know. *The Fenway Institute.* Retrieved September 14, 2014 from www.lgbthealtheducation.org

Bjorkman, M., Malterud, K. (2009). Lesbian women's experience with health care: A qualitative study. *Scandinavian Journal of Primary Health Care.* 27:238-243.

Bradford, J.B., Cahill, S., Grasso, C., Makadon, H.J. (2014). How to gather data on sexual orientation and gender identity in clinical settings. *The Fenway Institute.* Retrieved on September 14, 2014 from www.fenwayinstitute.org

Crisp, C. (2006). The Gay Affirmative Practice Scale: A new measure for assessing cultural competence with Gay and Lesbian patients. *Social Work.* 51(2). 115-126. LGBT Healthlink. (2014). Healthcare Bill of Rights. Retrieved on March 14, 2015 from www.healthcarebillofrights.org

Fish, J., Bewley, S. (2009). Using human rights-based approaches to conceptualize lesbian and bisexual women's health inequalities. *Health and Social Care in the Community.* 18(4). 355-362.

Goode, T.D., Fisher, S.K. (2012). Self-assessment checklist for personnel providing services and supports to LGBTQ youth and their families. *National Center for Cultural Competence.* Retrieved September 15, 2014 www.ccc.georgetown.edu

Graham, R., Berkowitz, B.A., Blum, R., Kasprzk, D. et al (2011). The health of lesbian, gay, bisexual and transgender people: Building a foundation for better understanding. *Institute of Medicine*. Retrieved on September 14, 2014 from www.iom.edu

Keepnews, D.M. (2011). Lesbian, gay, bisexual and transgender health issues and nursing: Moving toward an agenda. *Advances in Nursing Science*. 34(2). pp. 163-170.

Lee, J., Hahm, H.C. (2012). HIV risk, substance use, and suicidal behaviors among Asian American lesbian and bisexual women. *AIDS Education and Prevention*. 24(6). 549-563.

Lim, F.A., Brown, D.V., Kim, S.J. (2014). Addressing health care disparities in the lesbian, gay, bisexual and transgender population: A review of best practices. *American Journal of Nursing*. 114(6). 24-34.

LGBT Organizations Factsheet: After DOMA -What it means for you. American Civil Liberties Union - Retrieved September 14, 2014 from www.aclu.org/lgbt

Peate, I. (2013). Caring for older lesbian, gay and bisexual people. *British Journal of Community Nursing*. 18(8). 372-374.

Peitzmeier, S.M. (2013). Promoting cervical cancer screening among lesbian and bisexual women. *The Fenway Institute*. Retrieved on September 14, 2014 from www.thefenwayinstitute.org

Polek, C.A., Hardie, T.L., Crowley, E.M. (2008). Lesbians' disclosure of sexual orientation and satisfaction with care. *Journal of Transcultural Nursing*. 19(3). 243-249.

Rawlings, D. (2012). End-of-life care considerations for gay, lesbian, bisexual and transgender individuals. *International Journal of Palliative Nursing*. 18(1). 29-34.

Reygan, F.C., D'Alton, P. (2012). A pilot training programme for health and social care professional providing oncological and palliative care to lesbian, gay and bisexual patients in Ireland. *Psycho-Oncology*. 22:1050-1054.

Rew, L., Whittaker, T.A., Seehafer, M.T., Smith, L.R. (2005). Sexual health risks and protective resources in gay, lesbian, bisexual and heterosexual homeless you. *Journal for Specialists in Pediatric Nursing.* 10(1). 11-19.

Rutherford, K., McIntyre, J., Daley, A., Ross, L.E. (2012). Development of expertise in mental health service provision for lesbian, gay, bisexual and transgender communities. *Medical Education.* 46:903-913

Spinks, V.S., Andrews, J., Boyle, J.C. (2000). Providing health care for lesbian clients. *Journal of Transcultural Nursing.* 11(2). pp. 137-143.

Substance Abuse and Mental Health Services Administration. (2012). *Top Health Issues for LGBT Populations Information & Resource Kit.* HHS Publication No. (SMA) 12-4684. Rockville, MD: Substance Abuse and Mental Health Services Administration

Weisz, V.K. (2009). Social justice considerations for lesbian and bisexual women's health care. *Journal of Obstetrics Gynecology Neonatal Nursing.* 38: 81-87.

U.S. Department of Health and Human Services. (2012). NIHS 2013 Report. Retrieved September, 9, 2014 from www.hrsa.gov.

Suki's Story
When home remedies may not be enough ... | 11

Home Safety - Amish

Suki reaches far across the pot to stir the soup. At eight years old she is already quite the little homemaker, able to sew a straight seam and dust almost as well as her mother. As she weaves the wooden spoon through the vegetables she is thinking of her father, who seems busier than usual these days in the fields. He's the only one who calls her "Suki," a combination of her first and middle names. The first, Susannah, is for Inger's mother and the second, Karen, for his. Since she is the eldest child in the family, even though she isn't a boy, Suki has always had a special place in Jan's heart. Her mother calls her Susanna.

Inger has been a dutiful wife. She has borne four children after Susanna, all boys except baby Ilsa. The house always smells of lavender or fresh-baked bread. Susanna's smocks and the boys' trousers are always cleaned and pressed. Inger has never thought to question the "ordnung" forbidding the use of *electricity and telephones. Dinner is always on the table at five o'clock when Jan comes in from the field---even though the cooking fire is erratic and smoky.*

Today the potatoes in the soup, a sure measure of when it's done, are still not soft enough. Inger goes outside and checks to see whether Jan has begun to unhitch Alte. Jacob, her oldest boy, is with Jan in the field fetching water and learning how to motivate the mule. Her two other sons, barely out of diapers, are playing in the grass with the new pup. Only the girls, Susannah and Baby Ilsa, are in the kitchen.

As she steps from the porch Inger is seized by an unknown dread, a sense that she is not as perfect a mother as the Lord would wish. Rushing into the kitchen she is just in time to see Ilsa try to stand, pulling herself up onto the stool from which Susanna is tending the soup.

"Aaaach! Ooooh!"

Susanna's slender arms are flailing. Trying so hard not to spill on her sister she has dunked her whole right side in the soup. Immediately blisters are forming. The angry crimson of her forearm is in stark contrast to her pale legs and white apron. Susanna's left hand reaches instinctively towards the right side of her face, splashed from nose to ear by the scalding liquid. Just as instinctively her hand moves away as she rushes to the pump for water.

The boys, hearing their sister wail, are running up the stairs, but Inger automatically shoos them into the parlor, telling them to be quiet and watch Ilsa. Her mind is racing.

"I know it's not their job to care for the baby, but they must. And I must care for Susanna. Where is that salve Jan used for Alte's sore back when the harness rubbed it raw? Is it gentian that will lessen the pain? A licorice tea will help her sleep, I'm sure. Cold water worked well last time, when Jacob got burned, but that didn't seem nearly so bad; it was only his thumb. The mule is too tired after plowing all day to pull the wagon into Lancaster even if I could convince Jan to *find a doctor. It is his Suki though. We'll go tomorrow if she's not better---the whole family."*

Source and Safety

Oil and kerosene are the main source of light and heat for the Amish home. Cooking is done over an open flame. Open flames, scalding water, and combustible liquids increase the risk of serious burns to the children. Amish girls are more vulnerable to extensive burns and deeper burns than Amish and non Amish boys. They are also more likely to be on a ventilator for a longer period of time.[35] Therefore, it is not surprising that Suki reflects that statistic.

Suki's responsibility includes helping with kitchen duties, and caring for her younger siblings. While these tasks are familiar and commonplace for her, it only takes one incident to change her life forever. Amish girls are burned significantly more often from the ignition of their clothing and hot liquids. Home remedies are the initial treatment. Outside healthcare is sought only if it is determined that the healing process is not effective. Avoidance of "outside" technology is the guiding principle that influences their decision to seek healthcare. The Amish do not carry health insurance. As a result, hospital expenses are usually covered by the family and their community.

> *Reflective exercise: Health Beliefs & Home Remedies*
> 1. *Were you aware that Amish girls are at greatest risk for burns?*
> 2. *From your perspective ~ are home remedies indicated in this situation?*
> 3. *Did your family use home remedies and a "wait & see" approach?*
> 4. *Do you discuss the use & effectiveness of home remedies with your patients?*
> 5. *If you disagree with their methods, do you speak up? Offer alternatives?*

The Amish Story

Amish roots go deep. The tenets of their beliefs began in 1525 in Zurich, Switzerland, when a group of religious dissenters challenged the tenets of the Protestant Reformation. They were strongly opposed to government sponsorship of religion and infant baptism. The group came to be known as Anabaptists which correlates with their belief in adult baptism. Many were persecuted and put to death by a government which was aligned with the Roman Catholic, Lutherans and Protestant church.

Years later they split into two factions – the Mennonites and the Anabaptists. The Mennonites emerged because, in their opinion, the Anabaptist were not strident enough. Shortly thereafter, a third group emerged – the Amish. The reason? The Mennonites were not conservative enough. Due to each groups' unwillingness to bear arms, or to accept the authority of the state church in matters of faith and practice, they saw themselves as disenfranchised from the larger community.[36] This lead to emigration to other countries. Many Amish came to the United States. The reason – the desire for a better life, to own property, and to practice their religion openly.

The 1860s brought further schisms within the Amish community. Two groups formed – the Amish-Mennonites (progressive) and the Old Order Amish (conservative). Today there are multiple affiliations or fellowships. These include the Schwartzentuber Amish, the New Order Amish, and the New New Order Amish. Each group has a unique interpretation of their world. For example, the Schwartzentuber Amish do not allow members to attach the orange *slow moving vehicle* signs (SMV) to the back of their buggies, while the New Order Amish, a more progressive group and with an interest for safety, allow SMV as well as battery operated turn signals and lights.

Today the Amish reside west to California, north to Ontario Canada, east to Pennsylvania and south to Florida. Their population has grown from initial immigration in the 1700s of 5,000 to approximately 175,000 today. The majority live in the rural areas of Pennsylvania, Ohio and Indiana. The largest community is found in the Holmes County region of Ohio Appalachia.

Cultural Beliefs & Values

The culture and community of the Amish way of life is not influenced by the outside world. Suki's family are members of the Old Order Amish group. Their worldview incorporates an understanding of boundary maintenance between Amish and non Amish. Dr. Madeleine Leininger highlights that obedience and conformity to the community's rules of discipline are indicators of loyalty to God.[37] Listed below are some of the cultural beliefs and values that guide conduct, behavior, communication and manner of life.

Standards for Living the Amish Life

- Serving others through mutual caring
- Inner harmony by living a peaceful life
- Participation in activities that promote community well-being
- Religious beliefs and practices
- Separate from mainstream
- Follow the Ordnung

It is the responsibility of those living within a district to work together to ensure that everyones needs are met. Hierarchal in structure, each person's role is clearly delineated within the family and community. As a result harmony and balance are maintained. The rules and regulations set forth in the Ordnung provide the criterion for living the Amish life.

> *Reflective exercise: Cultural beliefs & values*
> 1. *Which of the cultural beliefs do you identify with most? The least?*
> 2. *Is there a set of tenets or religious beliefs that you ascribe to and follow?*
> 3. *What if you disagree with your patient's beliefs – how would you broach the subject?*
> 4. *Where to you find common ground to begin the conversation?*

Family/Community

Cultural values and hierarchal structure serve as the standard by which the Amish lead their life. The roles of men, women, and children are determined by scripture. They are not open to interpretation. Men are considered the head of the household and designated as the ultimate authority within the family structure. They contribute to the family by working the farm or seeking employment in nearby towns. Fathers serves as a role model for their sons. They rarely show or discuss their feelings. The mother is given a high status within the family. She is respected for her contributions to the household structure and maintenance. She is a role model for her children, primarily her daughters. She is expected to be submissive and obedient to her husband, especially in public.

Both parents share the responsibility of raising the children. Children are considered gifts from God. The average number of children per family is six to eight. This compares to a non-Amish family which is slightly more than two. Household and farm responsibilities are based on gender role and age. Boys apprentice in their father's trade. Girls assist with maintenance of the household and caring for the younger children. They attend Amish school until the 8th grade, and then graduate to a more significant role in the house or on the farm.

Elders are held in high esteem by family and community. Respected for their wisdom and life experience, family members seek their advice before making a final decision. They provide a strong foundation that promotes Amish beliefs and values. In their elder years it is common for them to turn the farm over to their sons and move to what is called a "doudy house" which is a smaller house on the property. They continue to be active participants in the family.

Visiting community members is an integral part of being family. Socialization is a highly held value, and families travel great distances to spend time with others. These visits provide an opportunity for women to spend time with other women in a relaxed environment, knowing that their children are enjoying their friends as well. For Amish men, this is time of relaxation and an occasion to discuss farming concerns. In addition, these gatherings serve as an opportunity to discuss the needs of the community.

Communication

Within the Amish community, Pennsylvania Dutch, Deitsch (Pennsylvania German) or Hochdeitsh (High German) are spoken at home, work, and with friends. Deitsch or Hochdeitsh is used in private prayer and worship. These languages are used to disseminate news orally. Children generally do not speak English until they enter school. As a result, English language proficiency may vary depending on level of education and occasional contact with outsiders. Amish refer to non-Amish as "English" as that is the language of "outsiders."

Not outwardly demonstrative, the Amish may appear aloof to an outsider. More reliance is placed on what is implied rather than said. Therefore, it may prove difficult for the HCP to grasp the full understanding of the message. It is important to recognize the value placed on restraint, especially in conversations with professionals. Eye contact with non-Amish people is usually avoided. While touch is generally limited, HCP are encouraged to greet with a handshake and smile. An Amish patient may appear less restrained and use eye contact freely during a one on one conversation with the HCP. Over time, as rapport and trust develop, more information regarding their home remedies and health concerns will be forthcoming.

Health Practices

The Amish have a holistic view of health and healthcare. Health practices and home remedies are passed down from one generation to the next, usually by women. Health equates to the ability to assume one's role and fulfill daily responsibilities. They believe that the body is the temple of God, and each person is the steward of their body, thus they are expected to live a healthy lifestyle. When ill, one must do all they can to return to good health. Their locus of control is rooted in family and faith. It is God who heals. Another strongly held value in the Amish community is the importance of being aware of the care needs of others. Care, expressed in the Amish term "achtgewwe," means that in order to serve, one must become aware of another's needs and then act by doing things to help.[38] As a result, individuals may not take care of their own health needs. Illness often results.

Healers, referred to as Brauch Doktor, are trusted members of the community. They are highly respected for their skills and abilities to heal. As with other cultural groups, and consistent with the Amish belief of caring for others, they do not charge for their services. Treatments can include massage, tea and other herbal remedies, and prayer.

As noted in the narrative, Inger immediately identifies the salve to use along with the recommendation to wait a day before seeking outside medical care. In addition to a wait and see attitude, limitations such as transportation and economics may also delay seeking treatment. While the Amish have the option to use the services of the "English" to drive them to the clinic, they do not carry insurance. To do so would indicate a connection to the outside world. Therefore, reliance on healers and home remedies is the first option.

Nevertheless, HCPs are held in high esteem by the Amish community. Choosing one is a serious decision. Family/community members and religious leaders seek HCPs who demonstrate respect and advocate for the Amish way of life. A knowledgeable HCP integrates folk medicine, seeks input from healers, and incorporates spiritual practices.

Religious Beliefs

The Old Order Amish believe in the strict interpretation of the Bible. Two scriptures lay the foundation: 1 John 2:15 which states, "You must not love this passing world or anything that is in the word. The love of the Father cannot be in any man who loves the world;" and II Corinthians 6:17 "but anyone who is joined to the Lord is one spirit with him," are the cornerstone to their beliefs and practices. Members live in accordance with God's will. To live simply and to care for those within the community is the foundation of Amish life and faith[39]

Communities are divided into church districts which are made up of twenty-five to fifty families. Each district is served by a Bishop, a Minister, Deacons and Elders. These leaders, chosen by the community, are male, unpaid, and without formal education. While there is no regional or national hierarchy, Bishops meet annually to discuss common issues. Biweekly services, which include sharing a meal and socialization, rotates among households. These gatherings may accommodate as many as 150 people. Twice annually the Ordnung is reviewed at a service. Any changes made require the unanimous vote of all baptized members, men and women.

Faith is an integral part of the Amish belief system. It is God who heals, and as a result, prayers and religious healing rituals may be the first form of treatment. The results of a study done on the spiritual healthcare practices of the Amish provided both expected and unexpected results. The study validated the Amish belief in the power of prayers and God's control over the individual's health. Listed as the top spiritual healing practices were praying alone, reading spiritual material, family activities and praying with others. The surprising finding was that meditation, yoga, relaxation techniques and exercise were healing practices as well.[40] The use of all of these supports the holistic belief model that promotes a sense of well-being, good health and quality of life.

Educational Tools & Health Literacy

Amish complete formal education at the 8th grade level. However, most health education information and consent forms, are written at a 12th grade level. As a result of limited literacy, misunderstandings can lead to poor health outcomes. Therefore, key factors to consider when developing a health education materials for the Amish community are listed here.

- English is not the primary language
- Minimal contact with those outside of community
- Hierarchal structure
- Reading comprehension
- Community involvement

Providing an educational tool for home safety must take into consideration Amish cultural beliefs, values, communication, literacy and community structure. The Pediatric Burn Center at Shriner's Hospital in Cincinnati took on this challenge. The burn center is the regional hub for ten surrounding states. Given the disparity in burn rates between Amish and non Amish children, the medical staff felt compelled to develop an educational tool to assess home safety. Their concern extended to those who were treated at home and may have died from their burn injury. They asked the question – What educational material is available to the Amish community? Is it effective? They found information pamphlets that highlighted such items as curling irons and crockpots – electrical appliances that the Amish do not use. There was a Burn Aid Booklet written by Amish for Amish, although they found it was not disseminated broadly within the community.

Medical personnel wanted to develop an acceptable *burn prevention* teaching tool specific for Amish children and parents. They knew that an effective educational tool must respect and integrate the Amish cultural beliefs and values. In addition, community input was integral to the success of the project. Therefore, they sought input from the Bishop, an Amish natural healer, and the parents. As a result, they gained parent's permission for their children's participation in the educational program as well. The team then collaborated with the Amish school teacher to implement the tool and to reinforce at school what the children were expected to learn at home. Together they created an effective tool that informed Amish parents of the potential risk for injury specifically for burns from open flames or scalding liquids.

It was a success! The tool, a magnetic board, depicts children in their familiar environment – a farmhouse, a barn and a workshop. Magnetic figures of household items were designed to highlight potential burn risks to children. A flame magnetic piece illustrated potential fire. A fire extinguisher magnet was in a designated place within the home demonstrating easy accessibility. Working collaboratively with the Amish hierarchy and incorporating the community in the development of the tool increased its acceptance and utilization.

> *Reflective exercise: You want to develop a program to inform the Amish community about one of the following. Who are the key people to collaborate with on this program?*
> 1. *Pap smear screening & mammogram.*
> 2. *The HPV series for girls and boys?*
> 3. *Vaccinations for their children and themselves?*
> 4. *How would you evaluate its effectiveness?*

Summary

To effectively serve the health needs of the Amish community, it is incumbent on us to acknowledge the importance of family and community, to respect their ways of living in the world, and to work collaboratively to meet their health needs and concerns. As we plan care, consider actions that embrace all three aspects of culture care decisions and actions.

Cultural Care Decisions & Actions

Acknowledge & Affirm
Support/Counsel from family and community
Care behavior/Roles/Responsibilities related to gender, age and role

Discuss & Adjust
Folk remedies
Flexible scheduling
Include family members

Collaborate & Change
Home/Farm Safety
Provide knowledge of human physiology

Resources

Diddle, G., Denham, S.A. (2010). Spirituality and its relationships with health and illness of Appalachian People. *Journal of Transcultural Nursing.* 21(2). pp. 175-182.

Donnermeyer, J.F., Friedrich, L. (2006). Amish society: An overview reconsidered. *The Journal of Multicultural Nursing & Health.* 12(3). pp. 35-43.

Amish Studies. (2010). The Young Center for Anabaptist and Pietist Studies: Amish population by state. Retrieved on March 3, 2015 from www2.etown.edu/amishstudies/Population_by_State_2012.asp

Gibson, E.A. (2008). Critically ill Amish newborn: An application of Leininger's theory of Culture Care Diversity and Universality. *Journal of Transcultural Nursing.* 19(4). pp. 371-374.

Gillum, D.R., Staffileno, B.A. (2011). An integrative review of the current knowledge of cardiovascular disease and associated risk factors in the Old Order Amish. *Journal of Transcultural Nursing.* 22(2). pp. 182-190.

Emery, E. (1995). Amish Families. In McGoldrick, M.M., Giordano, J., Garcia-Preto, N., *Ethnicity and Family Therapy.* (3rd. Ed.). New York: The Guilford Press.

Finn, J. (1995). Leininger's model for discoveries at The Farm and Midwifery services to the Amish. *Journal of Transcultural Nursing.* 7(1). pp. 28-35.

Kahn, S.A., Demme, R.A., Lentz, C.W. (2012). Mortality after treating severe burns with traditional Amish home remedies: A case report, literature review and ethical discussion. Retrieved on March 3, 2015 from www.elsevier.com/locate/burns.

Katz, M.L., Ferketich, A.K., Paskett, E.D., Bloomfield, C.D. (2013). Health literacy among the Amish: Measuring a complex concept among a unique population. *Journal of Community Health.* 38:753-758.

Posmontier, B., Horowitz, J.A. (2004). Postpartum practices and depression prevalences: Technocentric and ethnokinship cultural perspectives. *Journal of Transcultural Nursing.* 15(1). pp. 34-43.

Reiter, P.L., Katz, M.L, Ferketich, A.K., Paskett, E.D., Clinton, S.K., Bloomfield, C.D. (2009). *Journal of Rural Nursing and Health Care.* 9(2). pp. 33-44.

Rieman, M.T., Hunley, M., Woeste, L., Kagan, R.J. (2008). Is there an increased risk of burns to Amish children? *Journal of Burn Care & Research.* 29(5). pp. 742-749.

Rieman, M.T., Kagan, R.J. (2012). Development of a burn prevention teaching tool for Amish children. *Journal of Burn Care & Research.* 33(2). pp. 260-264.

Rieman, M.T., Kagan, R.J. (2012). Pilot testing of burn prevention teaching tool for Amish children. *Journal of Burn Care & Research.* 33(2). pp. 265-271.

Schwartz, K., Helmuth, M.R., Gillum, D.R. (2013). Amish Americans. In Giger, J. N. *Transcultural Nursing: Assessment & Intervention.* (6th Ed.). Missouri: Elsevier Mosby.

Sharpnack, P.A., Griffin, M.T., Benders, A.M., Fitzpatrick, J.J. (2010). Spiritual and alternative healthcare practices of the Amish. *Holistic Nursing Practice.* 24(2). pp. 64-72.

Wenger, F.A. (1995). Cultural context, health and health care decision making. *Journal of Transcultural Nursing.* 7(1). pp. 3-14.

Wenger, F.A. Wenger, M.R. (2013). The Amish. In Purnell, L.D. (Ed.) *Transcultural Health Care: A Culturally Competent Approach.* (4th Ed.). Philadelphia, PA: F.A. Davis Company.

Weyer, S.M., Rathbun, L., Armstron, S.A., Ronyak, J., Savrin, C. (2003). A look into the Amish culture: What should we learn. *Journal of Transcultural Nursing.* 14(2). pp. 139-145.

U.S. Department of Commerce, Bureau of the Census. (2012). *American Community Survey* Washington, D.C: U.s. Government Printing Office.

Harjit's Story
Please Let Me Go...
A Good Death

12

Hindu - End of Life

"It doesn't make sense. I've succeeded in every way I was told: Duke. UCLA med school, top of my class for heaven's sake, and then I became a surgeon; I should know a thing or two. My family shouldn't be so pig-headed about this reincarnation thing."

Harjit groans a little, intuiting his son's presence and perhaps his frustration as well. Of course the feeding tube may be contributing to his malaise, but Harjit has minimal awareness of it, having been unconscious since Tuesday. The last conversation he had been part of was Monday evening when the whole family gathered at his bedside in the Ventura duplex where he and Satma had lived for the decade since Ajay brought them over from Mumbai. His brother had flown in *from Cleveland, his daughter Jati from Silicon Valley where she worked with computers, and of course his beloved Satma and his eldest son, Ajay.*

Harjit seems to be dreaming. His jaw clenches. Ajay, still seething from Monday's discussion, watches helplessly as his father struggles to breathe. No one in the family had agreed with him last night, but he, as the oldest son and a surgeon too, should have the final say about his father's "condition." He cannot yet call it "dying". And Dr. Wilmoth, the Singh family physician, concurs totally with Ajay's viewpoint.

"Perhaps if we can get some nutrition into him he'll be strong enough for another round of chemo."

Satma, dignified and upright in a pale grey sari threaded with silver, waits outside the door to the ICU unit. Jati holds her mother's hand in solidarity. Despite her composure, Satma is amazed and angry that her son had seemed to provoke an argument about prolonging Harjit's life.

"How can Ajay not see that his father's feet have been testing the water of the Sacred River for days now, that it is the correct time? The stars are aligned. Harjit has said his good-byes, set up a scholarship in Ajay's name at UCLA, and now, just as he sets forth on a journey to a higher life, he is rerouted to the hospital. How I hope that he was already too weak on Monday to be truly incensed by his son's rash action!"

Reflective exercise: End of life discussions
1. *What are your wishes for end of life care?*
2. *Does your family support those decision?*
3. *Do you, your spouse, parents, adult children have an Advanced Directive?*
4. *Is this a conversation that you've been thinking about having for some time, but just haven't gotten around to?*

Cultural View ~ End of Life Care

In many cultures death is considered a taboo subject, believing that to talk about it is to make it a reality. In the Hindu culture/religion, death is thought of as a transition from one life to the next. Extraordinary means such as ventilators, feeding tubes, and pain medications that interfere with clear thinking, are considered intrusive to that process. Harjit and Satma do not want to employ extraordinary means as it prevents him from moving into the next life. Since Harjit had not signed an advanced directive, the responsibility to make healthcare decisions, in the Hindu culture, rests with the eldest son. In our narrative, the discussion between Satma and her doctor son Ajay portrays the generational tension surrounding end of life decisions. Ajay does not ascribe to this "reincarnation thing" and truly believes he should do everything possible to keep his father alive.

In the past, making end of life decisions, such as "do everything possible" or "comfort measures only" was at the discretion of the physician. Today we have availability of advanced directives to address that issue. But this was not always the case. In 1974 Karen Ann Quinlan, age 26, was brought to the hospital unconscious. She was placed on a ventilator. Her parents were told she was in a permanent vegetative state. They requested to have her taken off the ventilator. They were denied, as they had no "legal standing" to make decisions for their daughter. They filed suit with the hospital, and in 1978 the New Jersey Supreme Court agreed with the Quinlans. Karen Ann was removed from life support. A similar situation occurred almost ten years later, yet had a significantly different outcome. The case involved a young woman who had been in a car accident and was deemed in a vegetative state. She was placed on a ventilator. The Cruzan vs Missouri Department of Health case was brought before the Supreme Court of Missouri. The parents were denied the right to make the decision to take their daughter off life support. This decision was upheld in 1989 by the U.S. Supreme Court.

These cases were the impetus for legislation regarding end of life care. The Self Determination Act of 1991 gave people the right to make decisions regarding medical care treatment, and to designate a spokesperson if unable to speak for themselves. Ironically, twenty-five years later, only about 20% of the U.S. population has an Advanced Directive. Why? Much has to do with cultural beliefs, taboos preventing discussion of death, and religious preferences. Our narrative informs us that Harjit does not have an advanced directive, therefore his son makes decisions for him.

Hindu Religion

There are more than 2.5 million practicing Hindus in the United States.[41] Hinduism can be seen as a culture, a religion, and a philosophy. Individuals are believed to be manifestations of divinity with a purpose of self transformation. It is a belief system that began more than 4000 years ago. Its central focus is on reincarnation. Life is seen as transient and burdensome. Because of that, liberation from the birth-death cycle and entrance into nirvana is the goal. *Karma*, a key element in the life of Hindu people, centers on the law of behavior and consequence. Karmic thoughts influence one's approach to life and death. It is thought that one's behavior in past lives, as well as present, has both positive and negative consequences.

Positive acts lead to enlightenment and fulfill the obligations of dharma. *Dharma*, a social/ethnical code of conduct, has a focus on "ideal behavior." Individuals are required to fulfill their assigned role, which was determined in the past. *Dharma* is unique to each caste as well. Caste is distinguished by hierarchy, the color of one's skin, and is related to spiritual purity and pollution. It extends from the Brahmans (Priests) which are the upper caste and light skinned, to the Untouchable (handlers of slaughtered animals and garbage) who are considered polluted and dark skinned. While the caste system was officially abolished by the Indian government in 1950, it continues to be inferred in the home and family setting, especially in regard to skin color.

In addition to a belief in a Supreme Being or Brahman, Hinduism also includes gods and goddesses, each having a specific purpose. Shrines in the home include pictures and/or statues of gods and goddesses as well as candles, incense, fruits and flowers. The Vedas, sacred written scripture, include rituals, mantras, philosophy, customs and health practices. Unlike Christianity, Judaism and Islam, Hinduism does not follow a rigid doctrine or worship schedule. However, Hindu temples serve as a place of worship and the center of the community. They promote key teachings of non-violence (Ahimsa). Steeped in tradition and history, the Hindu culture remains faithful to its practices. Nonetheless, as in our narrative, we note that succeeding generations may challenge tradition and religious tenets.

History

Historically, the route through India was preferred by merchants on their way to China to purchase spices and silks. It is not surprising then, that over the centuries India was invaded and occupied by many groups such as the Persians, Muslims and Europeans. India was ruled by England for more than three hundred years. Through non violence, a tenet of Hinduism, Mahatma Gandhi turned the tide of colonialism to secure independence for India in 1947. It was through the legislation introduced by him, that the caste system was abolished, and equality for women and dark-skinned Indian people was enacted. Gandhi's philosophy of non violence and promotion of patience in relationships influenced many world leaders, particularly Dr Martin Luther King who led to the civil rights movement in the U.S.

The first Indian immigrants arrived in the United States in the mid 1800s. Initially working as laborers in the lumber mills of Canada, they later migrated to the West Coast, to work on the railroad and in agriculture. Unfortunately, as with other immigrant groups, they faced discrimination, especially during the depressed economic times of the late 1880s. Two legislative acts affected their immigration status. First, the Immigration Commission of 1911 which mandated that anyone native to India was to be considered Hindu. They were also required to pass a literacy test. Second, the Immigration and Nationality Services Act of 1917 excluded entry into the United States by persons of Indian descent. That changed in 1965 with the National Immigration Act which provided entry of East Indians equal to the level of Europeans.

Today there are more than 750 million Hindus worldwide and, according to the most recent census, 2.5 million reside in the United States. The 2010 Census report indicates that Indians have a significantly higher income, $71,600 compared to $57,000 in the general population. Their educational attainment level for both high school and college exceed that of the U.S. median as well.

Cultural Beliefs/Values

Hindu beliefs center around harmony and balance with the cosmic order, karma and dharma. This belief provides the foundation from which to draw wisdom and direction. These tenets extend into family roles and responsibilities, communication, healthcare practices and end of life decisions. Duty to family and caring for extended family provides stability and support during times of illness, disability and death. These core values extend beyond acculturation or length of time in the United States. While intergenerational tension may occur, loyalty to family comes first, especially when caring for elderly parents.

Cultural Beliefs & Values

Family & Extended Family
Interdependence
Harmony and Balance
Karma and Dharma
Education

Family

What traditional values are most important in the Indian culture? The belief in Dharma, with a focus on the social/ethnical code of conduct, dictates gender roles and responsibilities. Following one's dharma leads to harmony, balance and good karma within the family structure. In India, when a woman marries, she leave her family of origin and moves in with her husband's family. She is deferential to her mother-in-law and to her older sisters-in-laws. Her identity comes from her marriage. In this hierarchal structure, the father, or patriarch, is considered the primary provider and controls the finances. He allots a stipend to each son. Women are subservient to their husbands. As with most cultures, children are highly valued. Brothers have a genuine loyalty to each other, as well as a responsibility to protect their sisters. Girls are expected to assist with household chores. Both are expected to do well in school. There is a high value given to elders and those in authority. They are respected and held in high esteem.

Families may not adhere to their rigid cultural boundaries in public, but subtly integrate them into their daily life. Children are usually pampered by everyone. Their friendships are limited to relatives and family friends, rather than schoolmates. While many Indian women are highly educated and hold jobs, their husband is still considered the head of the household and the spokesperson for the family. However, we cannot assume that our Hindu patient strictly adhere to these cultural beliefs and values, or have adopted a Western approach.

In our narrative we see the dichotomy between parents and son – the strongly held Indian tradition by Harjit and Satma juxtaposed to Ajay's Western approach. Traditions, held in high esteem in India may not transition to family life in the United States. This can lead to tension and conflict between generations. Ajay, as the oldest son, has the responsibility to care for his parents. He is expected to adhere to traditional values of the home country. This presents a challenge to the HCP. Offering an opportunity for a family meeting may help facilitate a discussion and assist in the decision-making process.

> *Reflective exercise: Family ~ Traditional vs Western influence*
> *You ask Satma her opinion about the care Harjit is receiving. She looks downward. Ajay seems annoyed. Considering family structure, how would you pursue this line of inquiry?*
> 1. *How could you acknowledge and affirm each person's perspective?*
> 2. *How would you encourage input from Satma?*
> 3. *Have you experienced generational issues within your family?*
> 4. *If so, how did you reconcile the differences ... or did you?*

Communication

Recently I presented a talk to a philanthropic group entitled "How to Talk to Your Doctor." The presentation focused on various styles of communication and offered a practical approach to discussion about health issues with one's HCP. A woman in the group shared that her Indian physician "never looked at her" during the visit. From her perspective, he appeared disinterested. She thought, because he is a physician in the United States, he had adopted the Western value of eye contact with both genders. While she did not mention this to him, it did not deter her from addressing her health concerns. It is important to acknowledge that Western values such as eye contact or a hearty handshake are not always appreciated by those who've recently arrived in this country. In India it is taboo for a man to extend his hand to a female or to initiate eye contact with her. While eye contact is expected between men, women generally look downward when addressing a man.

Satma's and Hajirit's style of communication includes using soft tones, gestures and head movements. They may not speak of feelings or personal experience as that is considered too self-focused. Many are bilingual, speaking both Hindi and English. It is important to ask their language preference because, as we know, in times of stress, especially end of life, it is difficult to find the "right word" in English, when thinking in one's primary language.

Time orientation, for the Hindu patient, reflects the past while living in the present. A belief in reincarnation is ever present. Rebirth reflects one's previous life – good and bad deeds. Therefore, all three orientations – past, present and future – hold incredible value for the individual. Past orientation reflects traditions and rituals, as well as past lives. Present promotes living a good life, having good karma, and following one's dharma. Each ensures that the future life will be at a higher level.

Health Beliefs

Hindu health beliefs focus on having balance within the body. Similar to theories of the four humors, yin/yang, and hot/cold, Hindus concentrate on five elements that must be in balance within the body in order to ensure well-being. These include earth (bones, muscles), water (phelgm or kappa), fire (gall or pittá), wind (vayú) and space (hollow organs). Wellness occurs when water, fire, and wind are in harmony. Illness is viewed as deficiency or excess of any element. In addition to balance, Hindus may also ascribe to the ancient system of healing called Ayurveda, or "wisdom of life." The foundation of this belief is based on the three Doshas – vata, pitta, and kapha. It is believed these determine one's personality as well as one's propensity to illness. Both practices attribute good health to balance in mind, body, spirit, and environment.[42]

Furthermore, one's health and well-being may also be subject to nature or the environment. Karma, which guides the laws of behavior and consequence, could be considered a cause of illness. It is similar to the Western belief of cause (bacteria, virus, exposure to chemicals) and effect (ill health). Negative karma can result in illness as well. Moreover, external and internal elements increases one's susceptibility to illness. Internal conditions such as anger, jealously and shame; and external conditions such as affliction from the malevolent spirits of ancestors, god and goddesses, and sins committed in an earlier life may be the causative agents.

Healing practices

A study of Asian Indians residing in the United States found that 80% have a home shrine, 80% perform morning "pufa" (honour prayer) and 60% visit the temple weekly to perform a vrata, a ritual that provides personal protection and blessing.[43] Three main healing practices integral to balance, harmony and health, are prayer, pilgrimages, and astrology. Prayer provides protection for physical and psychological illness. Pilgrimages help to eradicate sin. Astrology is integrated into the previous interventions. Furthermore, spiritual rituals of chanting mantras, offering prayers to gods/goddesses and ancestors, ingesting holy water, and wearing amulets that contain sacred scripture are used to maintain well-being.

Ayurveda medicine incorporates herbal medicine, detoxification, and nutrition to restore balance and health. If the illness is believed due to bad karma, the patient may engage in rituals to invoke interventions by gods/goddesses on their behalf. Sacred scripture such as the Bhagavad Gita provide comfort and insight with a focus on self transformation. The ancient healing practice of yoga, which includes posture, meditation and contemplation is thought to have the ability to relieve anxiety, decrease stress and help one cope with everyday stressors in life.

Therefore, it is beneficial for the HCP to acknowledge the importance of balance and harmony and to provide opportunities for the patient to reflect on the practices he employs during illness. Those who seek restoration and balance in their lives are more likely to be open to interventions.

> *Reflective exercise: Are your patients more likely to rely on traditional healing rituals when they:*
> 1. *Live in a like community of culture and ethnicity?*
> 2. *Adhere to their religious beliefs?*
> 3. *Ascribe to a hierarchal structure with clear gender roles?*
> 4. *Respect their elders counsel and health practices?*

Healers

As with many cultures, family members, especially the mother, are sought for their counsel and healing powers before soliciting advice from physicians. Gurus, considered healers, weave divinity and traditional health practices. In addition Shamanic healers, Babas, Ojhas, and Jyotshis (astrologers) provide rituals such as chanting sacred verses or creating a talisman infused with healing properties to cure depression, ease anxiety, and reconcile social issues. Mystic healers aid with the spiritual side of self-realization or transformation through prayer, lifestyle change and meditation.

End of Life Care

In the Hindu culture, death is considered a passage from one life to the next – the process of spiritual evolution to enlightenment. The belief is that there is g*ood death* and *bad death*. A bad death occurs when a child dies, or someone dies suddenly and unexpectedly. A good death happens in old age, at the right astrological time, and at the right place (on the ground at home) with an opportunity to place holy water on the lips of the deceased person. Prior to a 'good death' individuals are expected to resolve any relationship issues (dying with anger can lead to a lower level of rebirth) and to provide gifts of money or property to family members. In addition, and equally important, family members and friends have an opportunity to visit and say their goodbyes.

The family makes decisions about end of life care. The question of disclosure must be addressed – do you tell the patient or tell a family member. The patient may choose to receive the information, or may select a family member to have that responsibility. End of life preferences focus on comfort measures, not extraordinary means such as a feeding tube or ventilator. Decisions regarding treatment or withdrawal of treatment for of those who are unable to speak for themselves are made by the head of the family, and in our narrative it is the eldest son.

There is a strong sense of filial duty by the eldest son. In our narrative, Ajay acknowledges this responsibility. Most likely he observed his parents caring for his grandparents. This current situation is an opportunity for him to reciprocate his parent's sacrifice and to demonstrate his loyalty to the family. However, Ajay does not hold similar beliefs about the end of life. He wants everything possible for his father. Satma, on the other hand, wants only comfort care for her husband. She believes Harjit has suffered enough. Suffering is considered a purifying and cleansing process to remove sins prior to death. It is seen as inevitable and viewed as the result of karma. Great value is placed on dying with a clear mind, not one clouded by pain medication. Satma is frustrated by Ajay's insistence on a feeding tube. Now, from her perspective, she believes that Harjit is suffering more than necessary. While she respects her son, she wants him to acknowledge his father's end of life decisions. Perhaps, an observant HCP will notice and bring about the conversation.

Summary

End of life decisions and actions are anxiety-producing especially when advanced planning has not taken place. The tension and stress can increase when culture and generational factors affect decisions and actions. Knowledge of the Hindu cultural beliefs around end of life and the ability to encourage this conversation must be considered by the HCP, pastoral care and social workers. This challenge offers an opportunity for family to discuss options and find common ground.

Cultural Care Decisions and Actions

Acknowledge & Affirm
Family loyalty and duty
Family decision-making
Hindu beliefs about end of life

Discuss & Adjust
Involvement in care
Mother-Son relationship
Family discussions & decisions

Collaborate & Change
Comfort measures for pain management

Resources

Anthony, F.V., Hermans, C.A., Sterkens, C. (2007). Religious practice and religious socialization: Comparative research among Christian, Muslim and Hindu students n Tamilnadu, India. *Journal of Empirical Theology.* 20 (16). pp. 100-128.

Ashurst, A. (2007). Palliative Care: Religion and Care. *Nursing and Residential Care.* 9(3). pp.113-115.

Bhagwan, R. (2012). Glimpses of ancient Hindu spirituality: Areas for integrative therapeutic intervention. *Journal of Social Work Practice.* 26(2). pp. 233-244.

Dana, R.H., Matheson, L. (1992). An application of the Agency Cultural Competence Checklist to a program serving small and diverse ethnic communities. *Psychosocial Rehabilitation Journal.* 15(4). pp. 101-105.

Datar, S. (2014). Grasping Palliative care. *Hinduism Today.* 36(1). pp. 58-60.

Deshpande, O., Reid, M.C., Rao, A.S. (2005). Attitudes of Asian Indian Hindues toward end-of-life care. *Journal of the American Geriatrics Society.* 53P(1). pp.131-135.

Firth, S. (2005). End of life: A Hindu view. *The Lancet.* 336: 682-686.

Gatrad, A.R., Sheikh, R.A. (2004). Hindu birth customs: Marriage, pregnancy and birth rituals. *British Pediatric Association: Royal College of Paediatrics and Child Health.* 89(12). pp. 1094-*1097*

Gupta, R. (2011). Death beliefs and practices from an Asian Indian American Hindu perspective. *Death Studies.* 35: 244-266.

Jambunathan, J. (2013). People of Hindu Heritage. In Purnell, L.D. (Ed.) *Transcultural Health Care: A Culturally Competent Approach.* (4th Ed.). Philadelphia: F.A. Davis.

Kemp, C., Bhungalia, S. (2002). Culture and the end of life: A review of major religions. *Journal of Hospice and Palliative Nursing.* 4(4). pp. 235-242.

McCauley, J., Jenckes, M.W., Tarpley, M.J., Koenig, H.G., Yanek, L.R., Becker, D.M. (2005). Spiritual beliefs and barriers among managed care practitioners. *Journal of Religion and Health.* 44(2). pp. 137-146.

Miller, S.W., Lass, K.A. (2013). East Indian Hindu Americans. In Giger, J.N. (Ed.). *Transcultural Nursing: Assessment & Intervention.* (6th Ed.). Missouri: Elsevier Mosby

Pillari, V. (2005). Indian Hindu Families. In McGoldrick, M.M., Giordano, J.. Garcia- Preto, N. (Eds.). *Ethnicity and Family Therapy.* (3rd Ed.). Guilford Press: New York.

Pennachio, D.L. (2004). Caring for Filipino, Southeast Asian and Indian patients. *Medical Economics.* 81(20). pp. 38-44.

Rambachan, A. (2015). The future of Hinduism in America's changing religious landscape. *Huffington Post*

Rao, A.S., Desphande, O.M., Jamoona, C., Reid, C.M. (2008). Elderly Indo-Caribbean Hindus and end-of-life care: A community -based exploratory study. *Journal of the American Geriatrics Society.* 56(6). pp.1129-1133

Samanta, J. (2012). Equality for followers of South Asian religions in end-of-life care. *Nursing Ethics.* 20(4). p382-391.

Sharma, H., Jagdish, V., Anusha, P., Bharti, S. (2013). End-of-life care: Indian perspective. *Indian Journal of Psychiatry.* 55: 293-298.

Sharma, R.K., Khosla, N., Tulsky, J.A., Carrese, J.A. (2011). Traditional expectations versus US realities: First- and Second-generation Asian Indian perspectives on end-of-life care. *Journal of General Internal Medicine.* 27(3). pp. 311-317.

Simha, S., Noble, S., Chaturvedi, S.K. (2013). Spiritual concerns in Hindu cancer patients undergoing palliative care: A qualitative study. *Indian Journal of Palliative Care.* 19(2). pp. 99-105.

Strada, M. (2001). Science, religion and ecology turn eastward. *USA Today.* 130. 2676.

Shin's Story

Can't you control your child? | 13

Autism - Korean Family

Shin is screaming. Hy knows that it will pass, also that she can do little to stop him. At eight years old he will soon be too tall for her to move physically. For now, even though they are out on a rare visit to WalMart for toilet paper and rice, she tries to speak in a soothing voice and direct him towards the door.

At the first scream Hy's mother, Hea Jung, has grimaced, looked around furtively, and headed for the restroom. Her grandson continues to embarrass her. Sometimes he wants to hold her hand as she sings the Korean songs her father taught her, but he doesn't ever seem to show loving respect for her grace and nobility; dealing with autism certainly doesn't bring out her strengths. Shin should be honoring her though, not the other way around. And here she thought Hy would produce a dutiful and brilliant grandson!

Shin's other family, his aunts and uncles and cousins, even his grandfather Bae, have distanced themselves from Hy and "her problem." At first everyone gathered for his naming ceremony, a special one for the first male child to be born in America. For his next couple of birthdays they were there too. Both Hy and her mother had high hopes for little Shin. Maybe he will go to Harvard and study medicine. Maybe he will be an engineer of great bridges. Maybe he will discover a new kind of technology. He will make the family proud. Here he is now in a special classroom---not special in a good way, one for problem sons. It does seem as if all his classmates are boys.

"So what happened?" Hy wonders to herself as she smoothes Shin's hair. "Why did he change? Was it something I did? I know that old white doctor at the clinic said "no", but I think he was just trying to move on to the next patient. Maybe if we had insurance he would have been able to help. He couldn't understand my English anyway, and he didn't seem to get it when I told him I was fine – though heaven knows Shin's strange behavior in the office shouldn't have needed a translator. He was screaming then too, I remember."

Out in the WalMart parking lot Shin seems to quiet. A blue Honda with its windows down has the radio on and the Chipmunk Song, one of Shin's favorites, is playing. Hy cannot look up to show her gratitude to the teenaged driver. Her whole body seems to shrink even as she holds Shin close. Mother and son will just have to wait for Hea Jung to powder her nose—as long as it takes.

The Stigma of Autism

Autism usually appears in the first three years of life. It is thought to affect the brain's development of social and communicative skills. The cause is still unknown. A report released by the U.S. Center for Disease Control and Prevention (CDC) suggests that autism and related disorders are more common than previously thought. It is unclear whether this is due to more requests for screening or an increased ability to diagnose the condition.

The stigma of mental illness has been deeply ingrained within Korean society for centuries and is thought to bring shame to the family. In our narrative, Shin has been diagnosed as autistic. In addition, he has a limited ability to achieve academically. This affects the family's sense of well-being, and is viewed by them as a portent for an uncertain future. "More so than other populations, Korean-Americans really measure their own self-worth, and the worth of the family, in terms of what the child is able to achieve and what the child means to the family," said Roy Richard Grinker, professor of anthropology at George Washington University.[44] For Koreans, mental illness comes in three stages: becoming alarmed, awakening, then acknowledging. Becoming alarmed by the child's behavior leads to awakening. It is only when the parents acknowledge that home remedies are ineffective that Western treatment is considered. [45]

Amy Lennard Goehner, who works with Korean mothers of autistic children living in New York City, notes that the stigma of autism within the Korean community "causes strain on the marriage . . . the subtle ways that they (mother and child) were shut out of normal social or familial encounters . . . and how they isolated themselves by retreating from invitations to dinner parties or play dates."[46] Family loyalty, participation, and achievement are core values in the Korean culture, thus feelings of shame, due to the stigma of mental illness, can lead to isolation. To understand the full complexity of this issue it is imperative that we as HCPs acknowledge the cultural and social backgrounds of Korean Americans.

History . . . in Korea & then in America

Korea, one of the oldest countries in the world, dates back two thousand years. It is bordered by China and Russia to the north and Japan to the east. In the beginning   Korea was aligned with China. However, following the 1894 war between China and Japan, Korea was given full and complete independence and autonomy. Ironically it was only fifteen years later that Japan occupied and colonized Korea. They prohibited the people from speaking the Korean language, barred them from schools, and forced them to learn Japanese. It was not until the conclusion of World War II that Korean independence was firmly established. It was at that time that emigration, specifically to the United States, began in ernest.

Although immigrant quotas still existed following the war, many war orphans and Amerasian children adopted by US families were allowed to enter the United States. Following the conclusion of the Korean Conflict in 1953, Korean women, married to U.S. servicemen, entered in large numbers. In 1965 an amendment to the Immigration and Naturalization Act eliminated previous quota levels, thus facilitating an easier entry. The United States, viewed as a place of socioeconomic opportunity and superior education by Koreans, continues to be a primary destination.

According to author Bok-Lim Kim, this increase of Korean Americans has made them more visible to the American public as a distinct group, different from the Chinese or Japanese. He states that "this has been an important change for most Korean Americans, due to their long-standing unfriendly relationship with these two countries. Koreans tend to view it as an insult to be misidentified as Chinese or Japanese"[47]

Perceived and real barriers

Immigration continues today. Koreans are one of the largest groups of Asians coming to the United States. According to the 2010 U.S. Census, 72% of Korean Americans are foreign born, consequently, they have "one of the highest levels of ethnic attachment of all Asian groups – speaking Korean, eating Korean food and practicing Korean customs."[48] These cultural values, however, lead to increased isolation from the mainstream. As a result, many choose to work in family-owned business. Even though most new Korean immigrants are highly educated, English language proficiency and the unfamiliarity with the American social structure (work environment) may not translate into well-paying jobs. The inability to speak and understand English and cultural attitudes toward certain illnesses such as autism, may also hinder individuals from seeking healthcare.

Cultural beliefs & values

Considering Korea's history and interaction with China, it is not surprising to discover the strong influence of Confucianism in the formation of Korean culture. Woven into their belief system are the values of social harmony, devotion, obedience to elders, guidelines for moral conduct, and ancestral worship. Koreans value group over individual, elders over youth, and male over female. This assures a harmonious and respectful environment. Moreover, educational competition, and the highly valued academic achievement for children, assures financial stability for the family and security for the aging parents. Harmony, the result of hierarchal structure and loyalty to kin, is the cornerstone of culture and Confucianism.

Cultural Beliefs & Values

Family Integrity and Loyalty

Kinship based Community and Social Relations

Education - Academic Achievement

Respect for the Elderly & those in Authority

Harmony within Family

> *Reflective exercise: Planning the initial encounter with the Korean family?*
> 1. *Which cultural beliefs/values would be the most important to consider?*
> 2. *Which do you think would be most important for Hy?*
> 3. *Who are the key persons to include in this initial session?*
> 4. *How would you acknowledge Hy's feelings? Raise her self esteem?*
> 5. *In what ways could you help the family to recognize their options?*

Family

The Confucian concepts of filial piety, ancestor worship, social status and rank, promote kinship in communities which strengthens family ties. Additionally, obedience, sacrifice and loyalty to patriarchal authority provides stability and harmony within the family structure. There are unspoken guidelines that are tacitly understood by all family members. For example, the term *Jip-an*, which literally means "within the house," identifies both family membership, values held, and traditions practiced within a particular family. *"Ka-moon"* means "the family gate" and refers to a family's standing in the community. The family determines what information is to be kept as *Jip-an* and what can be shared with outsiders. Unspoken boundaries exist to limit interaction with outsiders. It is not surprising, therefore, that the concept of *Jip-an* is widely relied upon in the immigrant community. Because Koreans attach shame to a wide range of problems, they are highly selective about what is revealed. As a result, it is a challenge for the HCP to solicit pertinent information. Acknowledging and respecting the Korean values of *Jip-an* and *Ka-moon* are the first steps to establish rapport with Shin, his Mother Hy and the family. Listed are some essential values to consider in order to provide culturally sensitive and competent care:

- *Individuals identify themselves within their assigned role*
- *Mother-child unit is center of Korean family*
- *Women are caregivers*
- *Family protected by male household head*
- *Respect for the elderly*

Bok Kim[49]

Parents are responsible to support and guide their children and to provide every opportunity for educational achievement. The father is considered the head of the household and the financial provider, while the mother, even if she works outside of the home, is responsible for the maintaining the home, raising of children and assuring the family's healthcare. Children are to respect and obey parents and elders as well as worship them after their death. The measure of self-worth is directly related to their academic achievement – educational attainment connotes status for the individual and family.

As noted earlier, 72% of all Koreans in the United States are foreign born, hence intergenerational conflict does occur between "Westernized" children and their elders who ascribe to traditional values. As a result, this can lead to role confusion and discord within the family structure. Nonetheless, grandparents are an integral part of family life. Many live with their adult children and assist with meal preparation and child care. Respected for their experiences, family members seek their advice on issues, including healthcare.

Taking into consideration Korean cultural values, family roles/responsibilities, and expectations of the next generation, a child with autism may cause additional stress for parents, siblings and grandparents. The stigma of mental illness coupled with Shin's inability to achieve academically, signifies a future financial burden to his immigrant family. Unfortunately, Hy may not avail herself of outside resources due to her limited English proficiency and the taboo of sharing this information with outsiders.

> *Reflective exercise: Family*
> 1. *Within your family structure are there certain issues that are "kept within the family" so to maintain "family standing" in the community?*
> 2. *If so, what could a HCP or social worker say that would make you comfortable sharing sensitive information?*
> 3. *Acknowledging the values of Ji-pan and Ka-moon, how would you incorporate those constructs into your discussion with the family?*
> 4. *Is this approach to the discussion with Hy similar or different from approach you'd take with your family?*

Communication

According to the American Community Survey 79.2% of Koreans living in the United States speak only Korean at home. Furthermore, 46.7% do not speak English well.[50] Therefore Hy's level of literacy needs to be assessed. A translator, fluent in the Korean language and knowledgeable about the culture, must be provided for every appointment.

The key to a successful healthcare encounter is incorporation of the cultural values – hierarchy, kinship, and harmony. *Kibun,* a Korean concept, exemplifies the ways in which harmony is achieved. The term refers to a person's mood, feelings, and state of mind. It is thought when one pays attention to their *Kibun,* and that of the individual to whom they are speaking, a healthy and respectful relationship is more likely assured.[51] This form of non verbal communication is so nuanced that it may be missed by an outsider. Comfortable with periods of silence, Koreans find that few words are necessary to communicate a message.

Additionally, an affirmative response of "yes" may actually mean "no." It is customary to agree so as to avoid conflict. Bok Kim Lim highlights another important concept – shame. *Chae-myun*, or face-saving, protects the dignity and self-respect of the family. He suggests that a patient may be less likely to reveal sensitive information if it means the loss of *Chae-myun*. He goes on to say that in order to respect the HCP, *Chae-myun,* may prevent them from correcting or disagreeing.

Age and gender also determine the use of communication variables such as touch and eye contact. Touching among friends and family is acceptable. In some contexts, the initiation of touch must begin with the elder, not by the child. Once touched by the elder, the child can reciprocate. Likewise, eye contact is used sparingly, or not at all, with those in position of authority or elderly.

> *Reflective exercise: Communication*
> 1. *Do you generally share your feeling openly?*
> 2. *Do you consider your Kibun and that of another before speaking?*
> 3. *Do you that is necessary? Beneficial?*
> 4. *Do you modify your approach when conversing with those of a different generation?*

Time

Past, present and future are part of the Korean lifestyle. The past acknowledges ancestors. Similar to many other cultural groups such as Mexican (El dia de los Muertos), Vietnamese and Chinese (Sweeping of the Tomb), Koreans show respect for ancestors by honoring them with an annual event called *Chusok*. Held in the autumn of the year, the family travels to the gravesite of loved ones with fresh fruits, dry fish and rice wine. Honoring the past generations assures protection and guidance for the themselves. Present time orientation embraces punctuality with appointments and work. However, for social events, it is acceptable to arrive within one to two hours after the agreed upon time. Planning for the future is essential. Having strong focus on educational attainment assures the stability of the family – socially and economically.

Health Practices

Balance, a theme found within the Korean cultural values, is the basis for health beliefs and practices. Illness many be seen as a manifestation of cosmic forces that are out of a person's control causing an imbalance in mind, body, spirit. It is manifested in the loss of Qi or energy. The amount of Qi in the body depends on the balance of eum and yang. The disruption of eum and yang causes the illness. Symptoms of too much eum (similar to the Chinese term yin which connotes cold/dark), creates problems of lethargy, while a person with too much yang (hot/light) may present as hyperactive. Cure comes by providing a balance: hot foods/remedies for too much cold and cold foods/remedies for too much heat.[52]

It is common for Korean Americans to seek the advice of family and friends before seeking professional care. Additionally, a person may seek out a shaman (mundang) to restore balance. Shamans are usually woman with the power to communicate in the spirit world, and the ability to perform cleansing ceremonies. In addition to a shaman, many may seek counsel of a fortune-teller to help determine the cause of an illness. Mental illnesses may be seen as a punishment for bringing shame to the family, disrespecting an ancestor, or causing disharmony in the community.

In the Korean community, any form of mental illness may be seen as a curse or an unfortunate occurrence. Autism, a taboo subject and considered *Jip-an,* may be kept a secret so as to avoid the shame that may befall the family. Furthermore, parents may be discouraged from seeking professional help for the same reason. Requesting treatment information equates to loosing family honor. The dignity of the family supersedes disclosure to an outsider. As healthcare professionals we must be aware of the taboo.
surrounding mental illness, be knowledgeable about Korean culture, and create an open and welcoming environment that encourages discussion and promotes treatment.

> *Reflective exercise: Health & Mental Illness*
> 1. *Acknowledging that mental illness holds a stigma in the Korean culture - how would you approach the subject with the family?*
> 2. *What if they deny there is a problem – do you change your tactics; agree with them; allow the discussion to continue and hope there is an opportunity to address the subject at a later time?*
> 3. *You are developing an educational pamphlet for a health faire in the Korean community on Autism*
>   1. *What important aspects of the Korean culture need to be included?*
>   2. *Who are the key people in the community to invite to collaborate on this project?*
>   3. *Are there leaders in the community that must approve of the pamphlet?*
>   4. *Where would you distribute the fliers? Who would you ask for suggestions of locations to place the pamphlets?*

Religion

Historically, Taoism, Shamanism, Buddhism, and Confucianism were practiced in Korea, thus all have influenced current social values. Buddhism, though not considered a religion but rather as a pathway to enlightenment, is a dominant way of life in Korea, and has one of the largest followings. Confucianism serves to promote the cultural beliefs and values of family – piety, respect for ancestors, and loyalty to community. The occupation by Japan in 1910 caused the practice Confucianism to fade. In the past half century, Western missionaries introduced Christianity, thus adding another religious pathway. Therefore, many Koreans who immigrate to the United States, use a blend of these traditions and beliefs. The hierarchal structure of the churches and temples serve as a base of support spiritually and preserve the cultural values of the Korean community and ethnic identity.

Summary

As HCPs we must recognize the Korean cultural beliefs and values of hierarchy, family integrity and loyalty, as well as acknowledge that mental illness may present as a taboo subject, not discussed with outsiders. While mental illness is a sensitive subject, collaboration with family members, shamans and religious leaders, provide the foundation to develop a plan of care that will fit with and be beneficial to not only Shin, but his Mother Hy as well as all members of the family.

Culture Care Decisions and Actions

Acknowledge & Affirm
Respect for family structure
Ji-pan & Ka-moon
Kibun

Discuss & Adjust
Assess Literacy level
Use of culturally & medically competent interpreter
Use eye contact sparingly
Save face ~ avoid shame to person & family

Collaborate & Change
Address stigma of mental illness
Incorporate shaman
Include community leaders

Resources

Baker, A. (2013). Working to Combat the Stigma of Autism. *The New York Times.*

Bernstein, K.S. (2007). Mental Health Issues Among Urban Korean American Immigrants. *Journal of Transcultural Nursing.* 18(2) 175-180.

Bernstein, K.S., Jypung, J., Lee, J., Park, S. (2007). Symptom manifestations and expressions among Korean immigrant women suffering with depression. *Journal of Advanced Nursing,* 6(4), 393-402.

Cha, C., Kim, E. (2012). Assessing the role of culture in Korean Goose Mothers' lives. *Journal of Transcultural Nursing.* (24)1, 86-93.

Cho, S., Singer, G.H., Brenner, M. (2000). Adaptation and accommodation to young children with disabilities: A comparison of Korean and Korean American parents. *Topics in Early Childhood Special Education.* 20:4, 236-249.

Donnelly, P.L. (2001). Korean American Family Experiences of Caregiving for their Mentally Ill Adult Children: An Interpretive Inquiry. *Journal of Transcultural Nursing.* 12(4), 292-301.

Donnelly, P.L. (2007). The use of the Patient Health Questionnaire-9 Korean version (PHQ-9K) to screen for depressive disorders among Korean Americans. *Journal of Transcultural Nursing.* 18(4), 324-330.

Earp, J.K. (2013). Korean Americans. In Giger, J (Ed.) *Transcultural Nursing: Assessment & Intervention.* (6th Ed.) Missouri: Elsevier Mosby.

Goehner, A.L. (2013). A Generation of Autism, Coming of Age. The New York Times Health Guide. July 3, 2013.

Im. E.O. (2013). People of Korean Heritage. In Purnell, L.D. (Ed.) *Transcultural Health Care: A Culturally Competent Approach.* (4th Ed.) Philadelphia, PA: F.A. Davis

Jordan, P., Sin, M. (2011). Perceptions of depression in Korean American immigrants. *Issues in Mental Health Nursing.* 32(1). 177-183.

Kim, B.C. (2005). Korean Families. In McGoldrick, M., Giordano, J., Garcia-Preto, N. (Eds) *Ethnicity & Family Therapy.* (3rd Ed.). New York: Guilford Press

Kim, M.T. (2002). Measuring depression in Korean Americans: Development of the Kim Depression Scale for Korean Americans. *Journal of Transcultural Nursing.* 13(2). 109-117.

Lee, E.E., Farran, C.J. (2004). Depression among Korean, Korean American and Caucasian American Family Caregivers. *Journal of Transcultural Nursing.* 15(1) 18-25.

Marchand, W.R. (2012). Mindfulness-based stress reduction, mindfulness-based cognitive therapy, and Zen meditation for depression, anxiety, pain and psychological distress. *Journal of Psychiatric Practice.* 18(4). 233-252.

Shin, J.K. (2009). Understanding the experience and manifestation of Depression among Korean immigrants in New York City. *Journal of Transcultural Nursing.* 21(1) 73-80.

Wallis, C. (2011). Study in Korea Pus Austim Prevalence at 2.6%, Surprising Experts. U.S Department of Commerce. (2012). Bureau of the Census. Washington DC: US Government Printing Office.

Yang, S., Rosenblatt, P.C. (2001). Shame in Korean families. *Journal of Comparative Family Studies.* 32: 361-375.

You, H.K., McGraw, L.A. (2010). The intersection of motherhood and disability: Being a "good" Korean mother to an "imperfect" child. *Journal of Comparative Family Studies.* 579-598.

Liliya's Story
It's Not My Job...
It's Yours!

14

Diabetes - Elderly Russian Immigrant

Even though Marina and Ivan try hard not to show it, Liliya knows they resent her presence in their five hundred square foot apartment. She should have stayed in Vladivostok instead of following her daughter Marina. Liliya had a good job at home---she can never think of Napa as "home"---and she really enjoyed managing the personnel office at the credit union where she worked six days a week. She does love telling people what to do, which job might capitalize on their strengths, which salary would be out of the question. She had no trouble in Russia being forthright.

As she enters the Bank of the West, trying once more for even a menial position, Liliya adjusts her sling-back shoes, pushes her recently dyed hair behind her ears, and extends a hand. The office manager is expecting her. There is a sizable Russian population in the upper valley, and Carol is hoping that Liliya will be like Lara in Dr. Zhivago; it is obvious that she is not. Liliya is overweight and overly forward, too much in several regards if appearances are to be believed.

"So I come for the job behind the table in your bank. I am head of office in Russia. I work with people. How much you pay for job like that?"

Having had her assessment validated---this is a pushy woman who doesn't even speak English---Carol makes an excuse after a minute to check on a car in the parking lot that has overstayed its owner's supposed bank visit. Liliya follows, though she resents the cursory nature of her interview and this young woman who doesn't seem to show any respect for her experience. Liliya hasn't even had a chance to ask about health care.

Dr. Appleby, Liliya's physician, doesn't focus on diabetes in his practice, but Liliya had gone in to see him the week before, after conferring with the kids about managing her glucose levels. The doctor had seemed nice, though not much of a talker.

"Dr. Karlov always told me exactly what to do at home, what new medicine was available, when to have my levels tested, what foods to avoid, what to drink if I was feeling faint. Why does this young doctor seem so ignorant of what I should do? This American dream is a nightmare."

Overview & Statistics - Diabetes

Diabetes is a metabolic disorder that occurs when either the pancreas does not produce enough insulin or the insulin available is not effective. According to the World Health Organization (WHO), there are 347 million people worldwide with diabetes. The Center for Disease Control indicates in their 2014 National Diabetes Statistics Report, that there are 29.1 million people, or 9.3% of the U.S. population, that have diabetes. It is the seventh leading cause of death. The cost of care exceeds $245 billion per year. It is most prevalent for those over the age of twenty, with men more likely to be affected than women.

Moreover, persons who are overweight, sedentary, and have a family history of diabetes are at a higher risk. While the greatest prevalence of diabetes is found in the Native American, Mexican American, and African American groups, Russians have the highest incidence within White populations.

Self management is the cornerstone of diabetic care in the Western culture of healthcare. Patients are expected to learn about nutrition, glucose testing, regulation of blood sugars and the importance of exercise. However, this form of medical intervention is unfamiliar to persons like Liliya who have recently immigrated from Russia. The method of care in the Commonwealth of Independent States (CIS) as it is now known, encourages trust and deference to the physician. They expect to be "taken care of," not to self-manage their condition. From a Western medicine perspective, control means maintaining a normal blood sugar. However, for Russian Americans, control means keeping the family together and ensuring prospects for upward mobility for the next generation.

> *Reflective exercise: 'Typical' Diabetic Patient?*
> 1. *Consider your 'typical diabetic' patient? Their appearance? Their attitude about diet & exercise?*
> 2. *Now add another dimension - culture and language.*
> 3. *How would this change your approach?*
> 4. *Does your current educational material reflect the face of your patient population?*
> 5. *What needs to change?*

History & Emigration

To understand Liliya, is to understand the strong attachment to her country of birth – Russia, the Motherland or *Rodino*. In the Tsarist time the emperor was referred to as *Tsar-batyushka* or "little father." From 1918 to 1991, the state assumed a "parental" role and encouraged social networks with family and friends to provide support for each other. With this sense of loyalty, it was thought that emigration to another country was equal to abandoning one's family and home. It is through this lens that we understand Liliya's current emotional and physical status. She may be experiencing a sense of shame for abandoning her *Rodina*. She did not want to leave her good job and dear friends. Nevertheless, Soviet law mandates that when families emigrate, they do so with all generations.[53] Thus when Marina and Ivan decided to emigrate to the U.S. "for a better life," Liliya was obliged to come as well. But this new life came with aspects totally unfamiliar to her – specifically healthcare.

According to the U.S. Census Bureau, Russian immigrants comprise ten percent of the foreign born population in the United States, living primarily in New York, California, Illinois, and Pennsylvania. While many are bilingual, the preference is to speak Russian. The majority are between the ages of 25 to 54 (47%) with the remaining 44% over the age of 55 years old. They are generally more educated; 80% have completed high school, and 53% have a Bachelor's degree or higher.[54] Though highly educated, their certificates do not always translate into high paying jobs. One significant factor is their inability to speak English fluently. As a result, they take menial jobs which lead to issues of poor self esteem, depression and family conflict. Liliya, would like to get a management job like she had in the CIS, but her inability to speak English is limiting her possibilities.

Obstacles on the way to acculturation

Liliya's loss of friends and employment, coupled with uncontrolled diabetes, may seem an insurmountable obstacle to overcome. While the dichotomy of life appears overwhelming, her sense of history, her values and her family provide the support she needs to adjust to living in this new country. In addition to barriers with employment, healthcare coverage is another impediment faced by Russian immigrants. Access to care can be limited by language, cost of medication, and lack of insurance.

In the Former Soviet Union (FSU), now referred to as the CIS, all healthcare is provided at no cost. The focus is less on preventative care and more on casual maintenance of health conditions. For example, a person like Liliya, with a diagnosis of diabetes, would not ascribe to a self-management approach to care, but rather visit the sanitarium monthly for her blood test and physical exam. The expectation of self-care, to her, is unfamiliar and unnecessary. It is the job of her HCP, not hers.

Cultural Beliefs & Values

"Cultural scripts" are consensually understood meanings and practices used by cultural groups. As a result, people from an ethnic group share an understanding of what is expected, permitted, tolerated and proscribed.[55] Understanding this concept helps us to acknowledge the potential conflict that Liliya is experiencing with her HCP and with her employment ventures. Cultural scripts and historical influences are integral to understanding the beliefs and values of the Russian people. Collectivism exemplifies the essence of Russian life. It is thought to be a response to spartan living conditions, harsh climate, or turmoil in government. Survival, therefore, relies on family and social networks. Collectivism, in the Russian context, is expressed as imposed social support in the form of encouragement and information regarding a health condition. It presents as unsolicited health advice ~ "you should do this . . . or that."

This counsel is viewed as a sign of caring and communal bonding – not intrusive. The pragmatic purpose is to provide "in your face" social support. Not asking for advice is considered a sign of a good relationship. Family and friends are expected to know what is needed, whether advice or action.

Cultural Beliefs and Values

Family & Extended Family
Collectivism
Hard Work
Interdependence
Education

Communication

Russian is ranked 15th on the list of languages spoken in the United States. Twenty five percent speak only Russian at home. Many elderly, like Liliya, speak both Russian and English. Effective communication includes direct eye contact, a firm handshake, and an appreciation for getting to the point of the conversation. Liliya's forthright approach – "So I come for the job behind the table in your bank. I am head of office in Russia. I work with people. How much you pay for job like that?" probably seemed aggressive and bold to Carol, the bank manager. Moreover, the meanings and sounds of words have a different implication based on one's tone of voice, inflection and flow. Pauses or gaps in the conversation demonstrate a respect for the wisdom of patience. Russians exercise less control over their negative emotional expressions with strangers, but more control with people they know. Positive emotions are more restrained.

Non-verbal communication may be minimal. It is said that following years under Communist rule, that to "look and act" neutral was considered the norm. Touch is used frequently with close friends and family as well as greetings with handshakes, hugs and kisses. Though a handshake with the HCP is accepted, further touch must be preceded by an explanation of the procedure or process.

Russian culture influences how a health problem is described and information is processed. For example, if speaking English, an individualistic approach using "I" and personal pronouns is used. However, if speaking Russian then a more collectivistic or "we" approach is used. In addition, Russians tend to use active verbs compared with English speakers, who use adjectives to describe emotions. Therefore it is vital to acknowledge that language switching, between Russian and English, during the appointment with the HCP can influence symptom appraisal and problem solving. [56]

Time Orientation

A "future within the present" a "present within the past" is the cornerstone to time orientation. To work hard now, and have patience so to suffer, ensures that future generations have opportunity. Punctuality is valued – arriving late is considered rude. The next generation is the hope of the future. Therefore, education of children begins early and is strongly supported at home.

Family

Families are close knit. Caring for elderly parents is considered a duty and responsibility. While Liliya appreciates, and perhaps expects, her daughter and son-in-law's support and care, she still misses conversations with friends and socialization at work. Both gave purpose beyond family. She realizes that her role in life has changed. Grandparents, like Liliya, represent the "old country" – a culture that may no longer be meaningful to the younger generation. Nevertheless, they are an integral part of family life. They help raise the children.

More importantly, they provide a foundation of security and connection with the cultural values and beliefs of the motherland.

Russian families may be described as matriarchal or patriarchal. Roles and responsibilities continue to fall along gender lines. Men are expected to provide financially for the family, show gallantry toward women, and participate in the decision making process. Women, as with many women today, maintain the household and child rearing responsibilities as well as work outside the home. It is not surprising, therefore, to see women in the clinical setting with multiple somatic complaints while dismissing any mental/emotional health issues. Similarly, spouses may limit personal disclosures to each other out of fear of "appearing weak." Therefore it is important to note that the HCP may receive more information if the patient is unaccompanied by their partner or spouse.

Parents take an active role in the lives of their children. They promote both academic and vocational excellence. Children are expected to do well in all things. Parents maintain an interdependent relationship with their children, yet encourage independence and self-sufficiency. This double message may be confusing for the child. Exposure to "Western" ways may increase that tension as they attempt to balance their new found autonomy and independence with the collectivistic/interdependence value of the "Old Country." Children may be called upon to be the "cultural broker" to help their less acculturated and limited English speaking family members to navigate the healthcare system. As HCPs it is important to offer certified Russian bilingual/bicultural translators.

Health Practices - Toska - Folk Medicine

Suffering, or *toska* as it is known, is considered part of Russian life. It is thought to have redemptive value. Hence, the patient may present with complaints of malaise, unhappiness, boredom and verbalize a yearning for the past. It is interesting to note that suffering does not carry a negative connotation. It is the belief that "everyone" is expected to have melancholy to some degree during their life. Therefore, feeling this way is considered normal. While the reasons given for the appointment are vague complaints of headache or fatigue, those same symptoms could represent an emotional condition. Unfortunately emotional problems or mental illness are rarely acknowledged. In the FSU, a person involved in unapproved activities or protests against the government was considered mentally ill. As a result they were admitted to a psychiatric hospital and given psychiatric drugs. One could be detained for several months to years. As a consequence, mental issues are rarely discussed and carry a negative stigma.

Health and illness are culturally formulated and managed by beliefs, experiences, and perceptions. Home remedies are passed down by grandmothers. Unsolicited advice is given by family members and friends. Russian Americans ascribe to both an internal and external locus of control. For those who profess a strong religious belief, illness is seen as a sign of punishment or a lack of faith – an external locus of control. By contrast, others trust in their inner ability to maintain good health – an internal locus of control. Traditional healers such as Znahari or Babki (old women) provide a combination of cures based on the symptoms presented. Home remedies such as herbal tea, enemas, hot steam, charcoal water or placing strong ointments behind the ear may be used prior to an appointment with a HCP. Medications prescribed by a HCP are viewed with reservation and concern about potential side effects. At the first indication of a side effect of the medication, the patient will stop taking the drug – and not inform the HCP.

Acknowledging the dichotomy of care provided in the United States from the "Mother country," Liliya expects a professional and firm demeanor from her HCP, someone who will "tell her what she needs to know and what to do." Her frustration with Western ways may appear as demanding and/or non-compliant. In the FSU, loud demands to receive care and magnifying complaints were the only way to gain the attention from the staff and physician. Therefore Liliya may display a certain persona in order to catch and hold the attention of her current HCP.

> *Reflective exercise: Health Beliefs & Practices*
> 1. *Do you think that we all have some 'toska' in our life?*
> 2. *If so, how would you differentiate it from a physical or mental condition? Or would you?*
> 3. *Asking "what they think about their condition" may be confusing to many elderly patients regardless of ethnicity. Are you comfortable "telling them what they need to know & do?"*
> 4. *Is there a way to include both?*
> 5. *Now that you have this information, what is the most effective approach you could use with Liliya?*

Diabetes Education

In our healthcare system, diabetic patients are expected to be participants in their care and to maintain a near normal blood sugar with diet and exercise. Self-management is promoted. A normal hemoglobin A1C is the reward for individual effort. However, for the newly arrived immigrant with diabetes, this is not the "Russian" way. In contrast to physicians in Russia, HCPs in the United States often refer patients to a diabetic educator for classes on diabetes, nutrition, and the importance of exercise. The patient is expected to attend these sessions and assume the responsibility of controlling their diabetes. This expectation is unthinkable to Liliya. She was always told what to do and never encouraged to be an active participant in her healthcare. How do we bridge the gap?

The American Diabetic Association acknowledges this dilemma, and has developed guidelines for cultural attentiveness. They suggest ways that a person's cultural beliefs and values can be incorporated into the plan of care. This includes referrals to outside agencies such as social services and mental health providers. For Liliya, it is more than the treatment of her diabetes, it is also about her loss of homeland, job and friendships. Eating a meal traditionally high in fat brings memories of the "motherland" and serves to maintain one's stamina. In the American culture, food may be associated more with emotional/psychological gratification or as a response to stress in one's life, rather than a vital necessity. Discuss with Liliya the foods she eats on a daily basis. Highlight those Russian foods that not only provide the nutritional value, but also prevent fluctuations in blood sugar, which can leave her fatigued.

Liliya does not like feeling "tired" most of the time. She may not comprehend the relationship between her symptoms and her blood sugar. This is an excellent discussion point and an opportunity to educate about the correlation. Maybe begin the conversation with this question – "What time did you last eat and what did you eat?" After listening to her response, suggest that you check her blood sugar. This is the moment to demonstrate the correlation between dietary intake and resulting blood sugar. Likewise, suggest that she do this at home when she is feeling fatigued, irritated or weak.

If her blood sugar is normal, perhaps you could include a broader discussion about other possible causes for lethargy, such as feelings of isolation and depression. Realizing that in Russia the physician also was seen to provide psychosocial services, this may be an opportune time for the HCP to set up an appointment with social services, one that offers translators and support groups for the newly arrived immigrant. While this is a complex situation, with many contrary aspects, incorporating Liliya's cultural beliefs, values and health practices into the place of care ensures good health outcomes – physical and mental.

> *Reflective exercise: Developing an Educational Pamphlet for Liliya*
> 1. *What cultural beliefs/values would you include? Words? Symbols?*
> 2. *How would you address Russian health beliefs and practices?*
> 3. *How would you incorporate "tell me what to do" juxtaposed to self-engagement?*
> 4. *Who would you collaborate with to ensure accuracy and poignancy?*
> 5. *Which person or groups would you ask to critique your finished product prior to distribution?*
> 6. *Are you writing this in Russian and English?*

Summary

Diabetic care management may differ from culture to culture. The HCP's knowledge of Russian culture, the significance of "Motherland," and the recognition of the belief in toska are all important aspects to consider when establishing rapport with Liliya. Encouraging her to ask if her daughter Marina could accompany her to the next appointment demonstrates an understanding of the value of family input. Providing information to her about community resources illustrates an understanding of her status and needs. Creating an environment in which Liliya feels understood and welcomed is the most important part of this process.

Culture Care Decisions & Actions

Acknowledge & Affirm
Family support
Working hard
Culture community/Religious community

Discuss & Adjust
Blood sugar awareness – signs and response
Use of non-directive approach
Non traditional health practices and healers
Bilingual/Bicultural diabetic educator/translator

Collaborate & Change
Eating patterns & portion sizes
Exercise regimes

Resources

American Diabetic Association. (2013). Statistics about diabetes: Data from the 2011 National Diabetes fact sheet. Retrieved April 23, 2014 from www.diabetes.org

Aroian, K.J., Khatutsky, G., Dashevskaya, A. (2013). People of Russian Heritage. In Purnell, L.D. (Ed.). *Transcultural Health Care: A culturally competent approach.* (4th Ed.) PA: F.A. Davis

Asfandiyarova, N., Kolcheva, N., Ryazantsev, I., Ryasantsev, V. (2006). Risk f or stroke in type 2 diabetes mellitus. *Diabetes and Vascular Disease Research.* 3(1). p. 57-60.

Barko, R., Corbett, C.F., Allen, C.B., Shultz, J.A. (2011). Perceptions of diabetes symptoms and self-management strategies: A cross-cultural comparison. *Journal of Transcultural Nursing.* 22(3). p. 274-281.

Bovovoy, A., Hine, J. (2008). Managing the Unmanageable. *Medical Anthropology Quarterly.* 22(1). pp. 1-26.

Center for Disease Control (2014). National Center for Chronic Disease Prevention and Health Promotion. National Diabetes Statistics Report, 2014. Retrieved August 22, 2015 from www.cdc.gov/diabetes

Center for Health Disparities. (2012). Russians and other immigrants from the former Soviet Union. Retrieved March 2, 2015 from www.iowahealthdisparities.org

Duncan, L., Simmons, M. (1996). Health practices among Russian and Ukrainian immigrants. *Journal of Community Health Nursing.* 13(2). pp.129-137.

Ehala, M. (2012). Cultural values predicting acculturation orientations: Operationalizing a quantitative measure. *Journal of Language, Identity, and Education.* 11:185-199.

Jurcik, T., Dutton, Y.E., Jurcikova, I.S., Ryder, A.G. (2013). Russians in treatment: The evidence base supporting cultural adaptions. *Journal of Clinical Psychology.* 69(7). pp. 774-791.

Kühlbrandt, C., Basu, S., Mckee, M., Stuckler, D. (2012). Looking at the Russian health care system: through the eyes of patients with diabetes and their physicians. *The British Journal of Diabetes & Vascular Disease.* 12(4). p. 181-184.

Magun, V., Rudnev, M. (2012). Basic values of Russians and other Europeans. *Russian Social Science Review.* 53(2). pp. 62-95.

Newhouse, L. (2005). Russian Families. In McGoldrick, M., Giordan, J., Garcia-Preto, N. (Eds.) Ethnicity & Family Therapy. (3rd Ed.). New York: The Guilford Press.

Shultz, J.A., Corbett, C.F., Allen, C.B. (2009). Slavic women's understanding of diabetes dietary self-management and reported dietary behaviors. *Journal of Immigrant Minority Health.* 11:400-405.

Schwarz, P.E., Schwarz, J., Bergmann, A., Hühmer, U., Bornstein, S.R. (2008). Perspectives and challenges to undertake diabetes prevention in clinical practice. *The British Journal of Diabetes & Vascular Disease.* 8(6). p. 295-298.

Smith, L. ((2013). Russian Americans. In Giger, J.N. (Ed.). *Transcultural Nursing: Assessment and Intervention.* (6th Ed.). Elsevier: California.

Stevens, J., Evenson, K.R., Thomas, O., Cai, J., Thomas, R. (2004). Associations of fitness and fatness with mortality in Russian and American men in the lipids research clinics study. *International Journal of Obesity.* 28:1463-1470.

Woldu, H.G., Budhwar, P.S., Parkes, C. (2006). A cross-national comparison of cultural value orientation of Indian, Polish, Russian and American employees. *International Journal of Human Resources.* 17(6). p. 1076-1094.

U.S. Department of Commerce. Bureau of the Census. (2010). American Community survey. Washington DC: US Printing Office.

Fusaye's Story
Meeting Expectations?

15

Suicide & Japanese Family

"If only I had listened more closely when Sharon told me of Richard's frustration. She should have known that my mind was elsewhere, that I was imagining how the cherry blossoms must look now at home. Why wasn't she clearer? A B in physics didn't seem that important anyway, especially when it wasn't a final grade. My children have always been so good at school, and Richard knew how Akira and I expected him to be an engineer. We spent so much money on his education at the university too. Why didn't he come to us directly? We would have listened..."

Fusaye, who is fooling herself a bit about her listening skills when it comes to her children, keeps arranging the teacups on the table. The university police contacted her at 8:00 this morning, but she can't quite grasp the idea that she will need one fewer cup. Akira doesn't even know yet since he's away on another pharmaceutical sales trip and she hasn't been able to reach him.

"How will I tell my husband that our only son, the reason for our struggle here in Seattle, has taken his own life? How could he do that to his parents?"

Sharon, who has heard about her brother's death but is still caught in a stage between anger and denial, has skipped work today to care for Fusaye. But her mother won't even look at her. Sharon resents Fusaye's quietness, her mousiness in the face of death. Richard was Sharon's brother too.

"Why doesn't she weep? Why doesn't she break something or slam the door or yell? Doesn't she know that Richard couldn't stand the idea of not measuring up to her nagging expectations, that he hated not contributing monetarily to our family while Dad was away for weeks at a time, that he loathed physics???

Reflective exercise: Suicide Ideation
1. *Have you, or someone you know, considered suicide?*
2. *What factors physically & emotionally contributed to those thoughts?*
3. *What changed your/their mind?*
4. *Did family or friends influence that decision?*
5. *Do you ascribe to cultural or religious beliefs regarding suicide?*

Facts & Myths About Suicide

Suicide is the second leading cause of death among Asian American college students ages twenty to twenty-four. They are more likely to think about, and attempt, suicide than European Americans and Latinos. Unfortunately they are less likely to seek professional help or disclose suicidal thoughts – unless asked.[57]

Suicide by Ethnicity in the United States per 100,000

General Population 11.3

White non Hispanic 13.5
African American 5.1
Hispanic 6.0
Asian/Pacific Islander 6.2
Native American/Alaskan Native 14.3

***Myths About Suicides Among Asian American**

Myth	Fact
Myth: Asian Americans have higher suicide rates that other racial/ethnic groups.	**Fact:** The suicide rate for Asian Americans (6.1 per 100,000) is about half that of the national rate (11.3 per 100,000)
Myth: Asian American college aged students have higher suicide rates than other racial/ethnic groups	**Fact:** Asian American college students had a higher rate of suicidal thoughts than White college students but there is no national data about their rate of suicide deaths
Myth: Young Asian American women (age 15-24) have the highest suicide rates of all racial/ethnic groups	**Fact:** American-Indian/Alaskan Native women aged 15-24 have the highest suicide rate compared to all racial/ethnic groups.

*American Psychological Association: Suicide among Asian Americans[58]

Risk factors for suicide, as identified by the National Institute of Mental Health, are depression or other mental illness, prior suicide attempt, family history of mental illness, chronic illness, family history of violence, and firearms in the home. Are these applicable to all ethnic/racial groups? According to the American Psychological Association (APA) the answer is yes and no. The APA cited research which found that while mental illness – depression and anxiety – is a predictor for suicidal thoughts in Asian Americans, social factors such as family conflict, viewing oneself as a burden to others and experiences of discrimination are risk factors as well.[59]

These findings are further divided into major, moderate and weak predictors of suicide. **Weak** predictors are immigration, acculturation and chronic illness. **Moderate** predictors include discrimination, sexual orientation, alcohol and drug use. **Major** predictors of suicide are anxiety disorder, depression, family conflict, and family cohesion.[60] When moderate predictors are combined with the major predictors, the propensity for suicide attempt increases. In Richard's case we get the impression that family dynamics, his perceived inability to contribute monetarily to the family, and the expectation to excel at the university may have contributed to his decision.

Living in two worlds – university and home – created tension and conflict with Richard's values. Asian American culture places a high value on family cohesion, harmony and interpersonal relationships, while the university values individualism and academic excellence. Nevertheless, researchers found that college age Asian American's suicidal ideation stems from the desire to die by suicide because of:

1). Perceived burdensomeness ~ an unfulfilled need to contribute to others welfare
2). Thwarted belongingness ~ unfulfilled need to belong to or disconnect from one's family.[61]

They discovered that a strong identification with one's own ethnic group along with family support proved to be protective factors against suicidal ideation and attempts. A positive ethnic identity correlates with a good self-esteem. The American culture values and elevates self-esteem. It is thought to be an essential element to assure success in academia, career, and relationships. This concept is used on many mental health tools to assess depression, anxiety and suicidal ideation. Yet, in the Japanese language there is no word for *self esteem*. Because it is weak or non-existent in the Japanese culture, the term should not be used to assess mental health. Therefore, it is imperative that assessment tools for depression must consider cultural beliefs and values, history, acculturation, generational issues and expectations of educational attainment.

History's Influence on Today

Prior to 1880 it was illegal for Japanese to travel outside of their country. That changed in 1885 when men were lured with the promise of money and housing of plantation work in Hawaii and the West Coast. Those who arrived between 1905 to 1924 came to be known as Issei, or the first generation. They were followed by the Nisei, or second generation, who entered between 1925 and 1935. Insulated and self-sufficient communities were formed due to language barriers and unfamiliarity with the host country.

In those initial immigration years, Japanese immigrants were met with prejudice and skepticism. On the West Coast, an anti-Japanese movement began in 1905, citing "unfair competition" and "lack of assimilation" by some of the residents of the communities. This sentiment transferred to the school system. The San Francisco School Board enacted the Segregation Order of 1906 to immediately segregate those of Japanese descent from the general population. Moreover, in 1913 the California legislature passed the California Alien Land Law which made those of Japanese descent ineligible for citizenship. They were denied the right to own or lease land. The law was upheld by the United States Supreme Court, concluding that it did not violate the equal protection and due process guaranteed by the Fourteenth Amendment. (Ferguson 1947 ~ California Law Review 35(1). The Immigration Act of 1924 further limited the number of Japanese persons who could immigrate to the United States.

The bombing of Pearl Harbor in 1941 proved to be a catalyst for further segregation and discrimination. Executive Order 9066, enacted by President Franklin Roosevelt in February 1942, changed the way of life for those of Japanese descent who lived on the West Coast. This resulted in the relocation of more than 120,000 Japanese to internment camps. Children born during that time and afterward came to be know as Sansei, the 3rd generation. Their parents "never talked about the camps."

It would be another twenty-five years before the voices of Nisei and Sansei were heard. In the 1970s, the Japanese American Citizen League sought an apology and compensation from the U.S. Government for those who had been detained. It took ten years before action was taken. The Commission on Wartime Relocation, established by President Jimmy Carter, found that the decision to incarcerate was based on "race prejudice, war hysteria, and failure in political leadership."[62] They authorized an official government apology, compensation of $20,000 to each surviving internee, and developed an educational fund to ensure this would never happen again.

Today, according to the U.S. Census of 2010, Japanese Americans comprise 1.3 million of the general population. The number of foreign born Japanese is 32% compared with the general Asian population at 74%. They have the lowest percentage of non English speakers compared with other ethnic groups. The Census report indicates that they have higher income ($64,000 vs $54,000), and educational attainment (Bachelor's degree 31% vs 18%) than the general population.[63] Their strong sense of family and loyalty provides financial stability and security.

Cultural Beliefs/Values

The constructs of Buddhism and Confucianism have a strong historical influence on Japanese culture. Confucianism promotes harmony in the social and natural order. Buddhism ascribes to non-violence, privacy, quietness and self-control. Together they form the basis for Japanese culture and ways of living in the world.

The first generation Issei held strong ties to the cultural beliefs, values and traditions of their country. The strength of those beliefs such as harmony, family, working hard, and mutual aid enabled them to withstand hardships, adversities and prejudices. Making personal sacrifices for their children was paramount to the success of the next generation. The Nisei replicated that belief and maintained strong family support. However, similar to other subsequent immigrant generations, the Yansei (4th generation) and Gosei (5th generation) have assimilated and adapted to the cultural ways of the dominant American culture. Consequently, the potential for misunderstanding and conflict between generations is inevitable. As we read from the narrative, Richard's desire to please and fulfill his parents wishes caused tension and conflict for him. How could he live up to their expectations?

Cultural Values and Beliefs

Harmony

Entyo ~ Non Assertiveness

Loyalty to Family and Extended family

Interdependence ~ Collectivistic ~ Group more Important

Honor and Respect for Elders and those in Authority

Politeness and Self-restraint

Duty/Obligation to Family and Work Group

Ambitiousness with Achievement

> *Reflective exercise: Culture & Stability*
> 1. *Which cultural beliefs and values provide a protective factor for suicide ideation?*
> 2. *Which influenced Richard to refrain from seeking help from a counselor?*
> 3. *Who could have he approached to discuss his suicidal thoughts?*
> 4. *Do your beliefs and values offer a protective factor against suicide?*
> 5. *Which influence your decision to avoid the discussion?*

Communication

From our narrative we note that Sharon resents her mother's "quietness and mousiness" in response to Richard's death. She wants her to be more overt – weep, yell, scream or throw dishes. From Fusaye's Neisi perspective, silence and restraint are the foundation she relies on when faced with tragedy. Would Akira, Richard's father, have the same response? Possibly.

Cultural values of harmony, respect and interdependence guide communication and establish an expectation of behavior. In addition, hierarchy, gender, age, marital status, education, non verbal behavior, and self effacement are taken into consideration with every conversation. Control over body language, limited eye contact and minimal touch are expected. When greeting one another the depth, duration and number of bows honors the status of the other person. While the Issei or Nisei generation may be more restrained, the Sansei, Yonsei (4th generation) and Gosei (5th generation) are more physically and verbally demonstrative. Recognizing generational differences in communication is a key to providing care that is consistent with Japanese culture.

Another aspect of Japanese culture is "empathetic identification." This concept implies that when a speaker identifies with views of the listener, there is an expectation that the listener will empathize with him.[64] Therefore, there is no need for a prolonged conversation. Furthermore, E*ntyo*, the cultural value of non-assertiveness, reflects politeness and self-restraint. It is used to demonstrate deference to others by playing down one's position. This conveys the ethics of Confucianism which gives thoughtful consideration toward superiors and elders. It may be expressed as a hesitancy to ask questions or to speak up in a meeting. Bringing attention to oneself is thought to show immaturity and lack of self control, and may bring shame to the family.

Each of these elements is integral to establishing relationships and developing trust. In the healthcare setting, the following suggestions set the stage for effective communication between the HCP and the Japanese patient. First, incorporate the value of empathetic identification by listening attentively to the patient's perspective – his/her viewpoint. Use eye contact sparingly to reflect their cultural value of respect for those in authority. An indirect approach may be preferable to a direct approach. Recognize that non-verbal communication is used minimally and does not indicate disinterest. Appreciate that the patient may sidestep confrontation in order to show respect and avoid conflict. As a result, nodding in agreement or saying "yes," may really mean "no." It may be helpful to offer options or ask the patient for their thoughts, before presenting the treatment plan or medication regime.

> *Reflective exercise: Communication*
> 1. *When you communicate with your patients, do you take into consideration gender, hierarchy and age?*
> 2. *Understanding the value placed on empathetic identification and entyo, how might you approach a conversation with Richard? with Sharon? with Fusaye?*
> 3. *Take the opportunity to practice entyo with a patient or colleague.*
> 4. *Did you glean more information about the person's concerns?*

Time Orientation

As with many ethnic groups, past orientation plays a part in everyday life. Japanese believe that ancestors have a responsibility to watch over and protect their families. Therefore, families offer daily recognition for that assurance. Moreover, a communal event, *Bon On*, is held mid summer to show their affection and gratitude for those who have died. Communities decorate and display lanterns, and perform dances to welcome the ancestors. It is an opportunity for those living today to remember those who've gone on to the next life.

Present day orientation promotes the value of harmony – the balance of here and now. Appreciation for the moment is not easily achieved as we read about how Fuseya is seeking peacefulness in the midst of her grief. Her display of a quiet demeanor is misleading. For her, losing control is not synonymous with her values of restraint and stoicism. The loss of her son does not bode well for her hope for the future, as the children, especially the eldest son is responsible to care for his aging parents.

Family

Core values center on loyalty, harmony and interdependence. Family obligation takes precedence over the desire of an individual. The patriarchal and hierarchal traditional beliefs held by the Issei, Nisei, and possibly Sansei. may create tension with successive generations who embrace the American cultural value of egalitarianism. Consequently, misunderstanding can occur within the family structure. Still, preservation of harmony, a core value found in the Japanese culture, maintains the family solidarity. The effectiveness of the family, therefore, relies on a collectivistic approach to meet their needs. This interdependence is manifested through the financial, social, and spiritual support that is expected to be provided by every member of the family. Problems are managed within the family structure. Interventions and assistance are expected and encouraged from extended family as well.

Traditionally families have been patriarchal. However, the role of the father today may be less authoritative as in previous generations. He continues to be the main financial support for the family. In addition to family, he displays a commitment to the company where he works and other collective groups. Mothers, many of whom work outside the home, are responsible for the maintenance of the family, child rearing and healthcare. *Amae,* the reliance on the benevolence of another, depicts the relationship between mother and child.

Children learn to be dependent on one another's goodness and kindness. From birth to around the age of five or six, children are given a great deal of attention. They are encouraged to openly express themselves. Permissiveness and tolerance of the child's behavior are expected. This all changes as they reach school age, when emotional reserve and self-control are taught. The purpose is to instill the value of obedience to authority. Education is considered the key to success and is promoted. The phrase *kodomo no tume ni,* for the sake of the children, connotes the sacrifices and hardships endured by the family to ensure the success of the children.[65] And it is the next generation who are responsible to care for their elderly parents.

Grandparents are held in high regard. They may live nearby or in the same house as the eldest child. It is the responsibility of the adult child to provide housing, financial support, and healthcare for their elderly parents. They accompany them to office visits to ensure an understanding of the diagnosis and treatment. It is important for the HCP to direct conversation to the parent, understanding that the Sansei daughter may intercede on behalf of her Nisei parent who presents a quiet and reserved demeanor.

> *Reflective exercise: Family ~ Family & Harmony*
> 1. *Where in the college setting could Richard have found groups of similar values and beliefs?*
> 2. *How would you introduce the value of 'amae' into the conversation?*
> 3. *In what ways is your family structure similar to Richard's?*
> 4. *How could you use that common ground to develop a plan of care?*

Health Practices

Beliefs in health and illness range from the Shinto religion, to Chinese Yin and Yang, to Western medicine. Some Japanese Americans may ascribe to all three, though one may be preferred over another. The Shinto religion holds the belief that people are inherently good and illness is caused by malevolent spirits. Purification rituals ensure healing. Yin and Yang, a tradition brought from China, focuses on the balance between the two elements. Thought of as complementary, and when in balance good health – mentally, physically, spiritually and emotionally – is assured. Yin connotes cold, female, dark, winter, while Yang reflects hot, males, light, summer and autumn. Descriptive terms highlight the components of each. For example, when a patient presents with somatic complaints such as fatigue or headache, and use words such as dark and cloudy to describe their illness, they may have too much Yin. Having free flowing Qi, or life giving energy throughout the body, is also thought to ensure good health. Qi surrounds one's physical existence and fills gaps between relationships with others. To make good use of Qi is to behave in a way that considers other's feelings and circumstances without displaying one's own emotions. Imbalances occur when Qi is obstructed. If flow is slowed or stopped, illness – both mental or physical – can ensue. Restoration comes from traditional practices such as acupuncture, acupressure and massage.

Patients are more likely to expresses somatic complaints of low energy (Qi) to describe their condition. They readily seek medical care for physical issues, yet are hesitant to address emotional or mental health concerns. Within the Japanese culture, mental illness may hold a negative connotation. Richard, strongly influenced by his Japanese culture, perhaps did not perceive a need for help. He may have considered his suicidal ideation a passing thought, and that he could improve his situation with herbal remedies. He would be more likely to seek religious or spiritual help, than schedule an appointment with the HCP or counselor.

Key factors to consider when selecting a therapist are gender and seniority. A therapist of similar gender with high seniority, implying expertise in the field, ensures a successful encounter. The therapist should not encourage the patient to verbalize any negative feelings about family members, because to disrespect someone brings dishonor to the family. Furthermore, some Japanese Americans are unlikely to assert themselves because of the elevated status assigned to their HCP. While the younger generation appear more overt and demonstrative with friends and colleagues, in the clinical setting they may appear reserved and passive.[66] To fully understand the health beliefs the HCP must consider the patient's generational status and their traditional folk practices and treatments.

> *Reflective exercise: Decision for Therapy*
> 1. *Have you considered counseling?*
> 2. *If so, did you hesitate scheduling an appointment?*
> 3. *How long did you wait?*
> 4. *Would you have considered a support group in lieu of a therapist?*
> 5. *Would you be more open to therapy if the therapist looks like you? Talks like you?*

Religion

The ideology of Confucianism, Buddhism and Christianity are intertwined in the Japanese culture. Ingrained in each are cultural values that influence behaviors, decisions and actions. Used individually or in conjunction with one another, each offers healing practices. Confucianism, with a strong emphasis on family, promotes harmony both in the social and natural order. The goal is to follow the tenets to ensure balance in all aspects of one's life. In the Buddhism belief system, the body and mind are one. The tenets of detachment, non-violence, quietness, reflection, and self-control promote harmony and peace.

Shinto shrines are sites that offer restoration of harmony through purification ceremony and rituals.

While the older Issei and Nisei tend to rely on traditional religion, the younger generations lean toward Christianity. A recent Pew Research study found that within the Japanese American population, 33% are Protestant, 4% Catholic, 25% Buddhist and 32% other.[67] Therefore, it is not uncommon for a Japanese American to be both Buddhist and Christian. On admission to a hospital setting it is important to inquire about religious beliefs and ask if they would prefer a visit by a clergy, a member from the Buddhist monk or both.

Summary

Myths and stereotyping that surround suicide may be just that – misconceptions. Nevertheless, culture must be taken into consideration when assessing for depression, anxiety, and suicidal ideation. Culturally aware and competent HCPs and therapists that are attuned to the nuances that underlie the true reason for a clinical visit are the most effective. For the Japanese American patient, values of family, the concept of entyo, health traditions and religion need to be incorporated into the visit and the plan of care.

Cultural Care Decisions and Actions

Acknowledge & Affirm
Family loyalty
Respect for elderly & those in Authority
Promote harmony
Hierarchy

Discuss & Adjust
Minimal eye contact & Social distance
Perception of mental health issues
Credentials of Mental Therapist

Collaborate & Change
Hesitancy to seek mental health treatment

Suicide Prevention Resource Center Terminology[68]

Suicide: death caused by self-directed injurious behavior with any intent to dies as a result of the behavior. The term "committed" suicide is discouraged because it connotes the equivalent of a crime or sin. The CDC has also deemed "completed suicide" and "successful suicide" as unacceptable. Preferred terms are "death by suicide" or "died by suicide."

Suicidal attempt: A non-fatal potentially injurious behavior with any intent to die as a result of the behavior.

Suicidal Ideation: Thoughts of suicide.

Japanese Americans may be classified into several social categories based upon their immigration, nativity, and generation history.

The categories are:

a. Isseis. They are the first generation of Japanese who immigrated here at the end of the nineteenth and the beginning of the twentieth century. Most of these people have passed on although a few remain. The Isseis were culturally Japanese.

b. Niseis (second generation). They were the descendants of the Isseis. They are American born and ethnically marginal between being American and Japanese (but really more American).

c. Sanseis (third generation), yonseis (fourth generation), goseis (fifth generation), etc. They are descendants of the original Isseis so many generations removed and most have little contact with Japanese culture and language. They have pretty much assimilated into American society.

d. Shin Isseis (new first generation). They are Japanese who immigrated to America after World War II. From 1924 until 1952 immigration from Japan was prohibited so this is the first generation of Japanese who came after WWII and are ethnically Japanese.

Resources

Alegria, M. etal (2004). Considering context, place and culture: The national Latino and Asian American study. *International Journal of Methods in Psychiatric Research.* 13(4). 208-220.

Brown, R.A. (2008). American and Japanese beliefs about self-esteem. *Asian Journal of Social Psychology.* 293-299

Cheng, J.K., Fancher, T.L., Conner, K.R., Ratanasen, M., Duberstein, P.R., Stanley, S. Takeuchi, D. (2010). Lifetime suicidal ideation and suicide attempts in Asian Americans. *Asian American Journal of Psychology.* (1). 18-30.

Chu, J.P., Hsieh, K.Y., Tokars, D.A. (2011). Help-seeking tendencies in Asian Americans with suicidal ideation and attempts. *Asian American Journal of Psychology.* 2(1). 25-38.

Coburn, C.L., Weismuller, P.C. (2012). Asian motivators for health promotion. *J ournal of Transcultural Nursing.* 23(2). 205-214.

Colclough, Y.Y., Doutrick, D.L. (2013). Japanese Americans. In Giger, J.N. (Ed.). *Transcultural Nursing: Assessment & Intervention.* (6th Ed.).

Ferguson, E.F. (1947). The California Alien Land Law and the Fourteenth Amendment, 35 Cal. L. Rev. 61. Available at: http://scholarship.law.berkeley.edu/californialawreview/vol35/iss1/4

Kawashima, Y., Ito, T., Narishige, T.S., Okubo, Y. (2012). The characteristics of serious suicide attempters in Japanese adolescents - comparison study between adolescents and adults. *BMC Psychiatry.* 12:191-198.

Kuroki, Y., Tilley, J.L. (2012). Recursive Partitioning analysis of lifetime suicidal behaviors in Asian Americans. *Asian American Journal of Psychology.* 3(1). 17-28.

Lau, A., Zane, N., Myers, H.F. (2002). Correlates of suicidal behaviors among Asian American outpatient youths. *Cultural Diversity and Ethnic Minority Psychology.* 8(3). 199-213.

Matsumoto, T., Imamura, F., Chiba, Y., Katsumata, Y., Kitani, M., Takeshima, T. (2008). Prevalences of lifetime histories of self-cutting and suicidal ideation in Japanese adolescents: Differences by age. *Psychiatry and Clinical Neurosciences.* 62. 362-364.

Pew Research Center. (2012). Asian Americans: A mosaic of faiths. Retrieved November 23, 2014 from www.pewforum.org

Selectman, J. (2013). People of Japanese Heritage. In Purnell, L.D. (Ed.). *Transcultural Health Care: A Culturally Competent Approach.* (4th Ed.). 218-233. Pennsylvania: FA Davis

Shibusawa, T. (2005). Japanese Families. In M.M. McGoldrick (Ed.) *Ethnicity & Family Therapy.* (3rd Ed.). Guilford Press: New York.

Shin, Hyon B. and Robert A. Kominski. 2010. *Language Use in the United States: 2007*, American Community Survey Reports, ACS-12. U.S. Census Bureau, Washington, DC.

Wong, Y.J., Vaughan, E.L., Lui, T, Chang, T.K. (2014). Asian Americans' proportion of life in the United States and suicide ideation: The moderating effects of ethnic subgroups. *Asian American Journal of Psychology.* 5(3) 237-242.

Wong, Y.J., Uhm, S.Y., Li, P. (2012). Asian Americans' family cohesion and suicide ideation: Moderating and mediating effects. *American Journal of Orthopsychiatry.* 82(3). p. 309-318.

Wong, Y.J., Koo, K., Tran, K.K., Chiu, Y., Mok, Y. (2011). Asian American college students' suicide ideation: A mixed-methods study. *Journal of Counseling Psychology.* 58(2). 197-209.

Theodora & Melina's Story Exhaustion! 16

Care Givers & Greek Family

"Ay, Mama. Would you stop with your whining about my weight?? It's too cold up here in Syracuse to walk and my back hurts anyway. Henry doesn't mind. When he's home from the grocery store all he does is sit on the couch too. If you want to complain, maybe you should have stayed in Greece. They have a Syracuse there too, you know."

"Melina, I'm not carping at you," Theodora offers in a melodic but subdued murmur. She has been cautioned by her daughter not to lean so far forward when she speaks or to move her arms. It isn't American. Her Greek is still totally fluent and will remain so until she dies, she knows. Maybe leaving her homeland at 78 wasn't such a bright idea, but with the death of Adrianos and hopes to be a real "nouna" in New York she gave in to Melina's urging. At least before she came over, her daughter showed appropriate "philotimo," what seemed like true honoring and respect. But maybe it was just obligation...

Theodora was delighted at first to see the priests from St. Gregory's walk by with their greying beards and kind demeanor. The nuns too from oldest to youngest were comforting and warm, though the real novices could hardly speak Greek. Maybe they are Russian.

In any case Theodora felt that she belonged there in St. Gregory's, surrounded by gold and icons and incense. "Melina is even a little displeased with my altar in the corner of the bedroom she chose for me in her home. How can I make sure she loses weight and stops smoking on the back porch if I can't pray comfortably in my own room?"

Melina, although she loves her mother deeply, has been hesitant to take her to see Dr. Philodokos even though he supposedly speaks a little Greek. Melina knows she is overweight. She knows her back pain and knee pain will not improve by themselves. And she knows as well that her mother needs to have a sleep test; even from her room down the hall Melina can hear Theodora gasping for air time and again every night. The doctor Melina had seen last year for similar symptoms had told her first to lose weight and then they'd see about that CPAP gadget.

"If he's sent my files over to Dr. Philodokos, I'll just die. Mama won't mind if we don't go soon. I'll buy some baklava at Gyro's as a treat instead."

The Unfamiliar Home

Our story begins with a life changing decision to emigrate to the United States. Theodora's ways of living in the Greek world have always provided her a sense of place and familiarity. Having family and friends close by – people who know what it means to be Greek – is important to her. However, the pleas from her daughter to move to New York are tugging at her heart. Melina assures her mother that she will "feel right at home" since there a large Greek community and a Greek Orthodox church nearby. For Theodora being a "nouna" and spending time with her grandchildren made the decision easy. She knew from conversations with Melina that her grandchildren are "Americanized," so she saw this as her opportunity to teach them about Greek cultural beliefs and values. Her decision to move to America was made with confidence in herself and her heritage. Yet, she did not consider the challenge of adapting to a new way of life and culture.

According to the social adaptation theory, the path to cultural adjustment to the American way of life is dependent on an immigrant's skills, resources, and social networks. There are three contrasting assimilation paths Theodora could take to ensure smooth integration: 1). traditional assimilation, 2). assimilate to the underclass, and 3). preserve one's culture and engage in the larger community.[69] On the first path, traditional assimilation, an individual becomes fully Americanized with a focus on socioeconomic stability and upward mobility. At age 78, Theodora is not likely to take this path. She has neither the desire, nor the resources and time to pursue such an approach. The second option, assimilation into the urban underclass, unfortunately leads to downward mobility and permanent poverty. Theodora has family and resources, thus it is not a consideration for her. Lastly, she could preserve her culture and engage in the broader community. This assumes a dual assimilation, one that includes both cultures - Greek and American. Theodora does not have to give up one culture for another, but embrace both.

History & Immigration

Greeks emigrated to the United States for one reason – the promise of prosperity. The first wave of immigrants came between 1890 and 1920. They were farmers, mostly young men. The impetus for coming was crop failure in their homeland. They came with the thought of earning money, and then returning home to buy land. A second smaller group came in the mid to late 1940s following destruction of property from World War II. The four years of civil war that followed left many destitute, thus the driving force for emigration. Most of those who came were uneducated with minimal skills. Making a new life for themselves was rigorous and back breaking. In 1965 The Immigration and Nationality Act lifted previous quotas and opened the door to those seeking life in the United States. Most of those who came during this third wave were families with children. They were more educated and skilled. As with previous groups, the plan was to secure an education for their children, earn money, and return to Greece to start a business. Most stayed. Belief in their Greek heritage, culture, and traditions provided the foundation and confidence to remain.

> *Reflective exercise: New Immigrants*
> 1. *Were you or your family of origin immigrants at one time? If so, why did they come?*
> 2. *What is Theodora's most pressing need? Physically, mentally, spiritually?*
> 3. *Do you think Melina anticipated the amount of disruption to her daily life that her mother's presence would create?*
> 4. *Have you ever had a relative come to live with you? Someone who was your elder?*
> 5. *How did that change your life?*

Cultural Beliefs and Values

Theodora's reliance on her Greek ways of living in the world provides her the self-assurance to face the daily unexpected challenges in her new life. However, it is difficult for her to witness the change she sees in her daughter. In Theodora's mind, Melina has given up the "old ways" for this new life. Although she loves her grandchildren, they seem to be caught up in this new world as well. Their friends appear more important than family which is contrary to the "Greek" way of thinking and doing. Greek culture, age, gender, socioeconomic status and education level guides Theodora's decisions and actions. Melina sees her mother as "old school." Nonetheless, there are core values on which Theodora and Melina have strong agreement: the importance of family, community, religious beliefs/practices, education/achievement and respect for elders.

Individuals are encouraged to take pride and honor in their relationships with family members and the larger Greek community. Philotimo, a Greek word that connotes the core values of honor and respect, reflects the obligation each person has to preserve personal and family honor. Creating a friendly and welcoming home, and showing concern for others exemplifies these values. Listed are the principle values for Greek culture.

Cultural Beliefs & Values

Philotimo – Honor and Respect
Family - Responsibility & Obligation
Respect & Promote Cultural Heritage
Uphold (Maintain) Religious Beliefs/Practices
Education & Achievement
Respect for the Elderly

> *Reflective exercise: Cultural Beliefs*
> 1. *Which of Theodora's cultural beliefs promote active participation in health and wellness?*
> 2. *Which allows her to let life take its course?*
> 3. *Which could you use to promote adherence to a health program?*
> 4. *Are your values/beliefs similar to or different than Theodora's?*
> 5. *Is there common ground to begin the dialogue?*

Family - Roles & Responsibility

Prior to her father's death two years ago, Melina rarely visited her parents. The geographical distance and the influence of the American culture had a curious impact on their relationship. Nonetheless, she knew, that as the eldest daughter, it was her responsibility to care for her mother. Loyalty to family and sacrificing for one another are tacitly expected.

Greek families ascribe to traditional and well defined roles and responsibilities. One is expected to defer to the greater needs of the family, and not place themselves above one another. The core value *philotimi* is at the center of all interactions. Family is considered the primary unit. Extended family comprises those related by blood as well as those with whom there is a strong relationship. Hierarchical structure ensures clear delineation between gender and age, thus establishing a cohesive interaction between members. There is a mutual commitment by the parents to raise the children and instill Greek culture and values.

Patriarchal in nature, the father is responsible for economic stability. While he may seem aloof or emotionally unpredictable, he is shown respect by all members of the family. Considered head of the household, he is the decision spokesperson. The wife may defer to her husband in public, however, in the home environment, her voice is integral to decisions regarding education, health, and social situations. A Greek mothers' responsibility lies in the care and rearing of her children. She, along with the grandparents, are responsible for passing on their Greek values, traditions, practices, and most importantly, the Greek language. Learning the language is believed to promote pride in their heritage. Many children attend school on Saturdays to learn the language and the culture. While the mother is nurturing to all her children, she may appear to be overly ambitious for her sons.

Children receive a great deal of attention and adoration. They are taught to be attentive during discussions, especially with their elders. Respect for and obedience to their parents and grandparents is ingrained at an early age. As with most cultural groups, education and socioeconomic achievement are strongly held values. Boys are presumed to exceed their father's accomplishments. Although a career outside of the household is considered unnecessary for the girls, they are expected to do well in school. Both boys and girls are expected to remain at home until marriage.

With succeeding generations, though, there is potential for intergenerational conflict. As we read in the narrative, it is difficult for Theodora to understand and accept the behavior of her grandchildren, especially their "American" ways. She does not think they show the respect for their parents or for her as they would if they lived in Greece. Grandparents and elders are held in high esteem and are known in the Greek community for their good deeds and community spirit. They are expected to participate fully in the activities of the family. In old age, and especially if widowed as with Theodora, their grown children are expected to care for them. If not, it may bring dishonor on the adult son or daughter.

Communication

High context? Low Context? Contingent on the style of communication, messages can be misunderstood in the process. North Americans, Germans and those from some Scandinavian countries use *low context,* while Greeks, Brazilians, and Italians use *high context.* How do they compare? Low context is individualistic, action oriented, and linear. Logic, directness, and facts are essential to the conversation. Straightforward and concise are necessary for a good conversation. In contrast, *High context,* considered collectivistic in nature, is intuitive, contemplative, and expressive. The message conveyed is shaped by feelings. Additionally, it is influenced by closeness and trust in relationships.

For Greeks, the focus is not so much on the words, but rather the context in which the message is conveyed. The listener is expected to be attentive and read between the lines. Indirectness is valued. Furthermore, their style may appear loud and overly effusive to an outsider. Emotions are shown by facial expressions, gestures and touch. Interruptions are common. There is a sign of engagement as one surmises what another is going to say. Eye contact is viewed as personal empowerment and connection. To sway one's eyesight away is considered rude. Touching and close use of space is expected. As a HCP, you may find yourself moving backward, but try to stay in one place!

Greek communication is considered warm, friendly and open. On a first visit, it is important for Theodora's HCP to create a welcoming environment that demonstrates an openness to conversation. A smile and handshake are well received. Showing respect at the beginning of the visit by addressing the elderly, with their title followed by their name is a key to setting the stage for a successful visit. Titles of respect may include: Kyria (Mrs.), or Kyrie (Mr.). In an attempt to avoid conflict or display a lack of understanding, Theodora may nod with agreement. Be aware that the Greek word "nay," sounds like a "no" answer, yet means yes.

> *Reflective exercise: Communication*
> 1. *Are you a High or Low context person? Could you change your approach if your patient were the opposite?*
> 2. *How comfortable are you with interruptions?*
> 3. *How could you use Theodora's effusive communication to your advantage?*
> 4. *Now that you have this information, would you approach care differently?*

Time Orientation

Past, present, future are all part of Greek time orientation. The past perpetuates and celebrates Greek history and culture. Present time orientation, while not always "clock oriented," acknowledges the importance of family and the "here and now." Future relates to the value placed on educational attainment and socioeconomic achievement, especially for the children. Parents will sacrifice everything to assure that their children accomplish their goals.

Health Practices

Theodora believes that "to be healthy is to have no pain and to take care of my family." In the Greek culture, health is a state of well-being, the ability to fulfill one's role in life, to solve one's problems, and of course, to be free from pain. Eating well, exercising and going to work are thought to be protective factors. Illness is thought to be caused by pathogens (bacteria/virus). Additionally, ill health is believed to arise from a more personal nature such as a punishment from God, a result of bad behavior, the entrance of evil spirits into the body, and the ubiquitous "evil eye." Wearing beads, especially blue beads, is thought to protect an individual from the "evil eye."

The "evil eye," found in many parts of the world, and in many cultures, points to envy, malice or pride. Known in the Greek community as *Matiasma or Vaskania,* it is thought to be the result of excessive admiration or envy from another person. Therefore, the patient is considered the "victim," implying one did not deserve or cause this illness. Children are especially vulnerable. Symptoms include vague complaints of fatigue, irritability and restlessness. Treatment options include making the sign of the cross over a glass of water, praying, and a visit by the Orthodox priest to rid the person of the evil eye. A magissa, or woman healer, may also be called on to cure the "evil eye." Thus it is important for the HCP to know that illness may not be within the individual's control. The belief in both the internal and external locus of control provides the context with which the cause of the illness is viewed.

It is commonly thought in the Greek culture, that stress leads to illness. Symptoms may be expressed as feelings of pressure. Three terms are used to illustrate the symptoms of stress. *Stenochoria* is described by patients as a feeling of being "squeezed into a narrow space." *Varostostethos* feels like a "weight on one's chest." *Anghos* is a "sensation of a choking feeling, as having a noose around one's neck."[70] Stress may also be equated to emotional or mental problems which unfortunately, carries a huge stigma. It is rarely acknowledged or discussed. Diagnosis brings shame to the family. As a result the person may become isolated from the larger community. Therefore patients may present with somatic complaints such as dizziness, fatigue, numbness in extremities, headache and backache. Feelings of depression or anxiety are kept in reserve.

Melina realizes that she is short tempered and less tolerant of her mother's many requests. "All she really wants is a good night's sleep and to wake up pain free and feeling happy again." There doesn't seem to be anyone to help or provide respite. Her friends are busy with their families. Her husband is hard at work at the grocery store. The children are occupied with school and church activities. The responsibility to care for her mother falls to her alone. At her last clinic visit, she tried talking with her HCP. It was not a good experience. From her perspective, he was dismissive of her concerns. The counsel was the same – stop smoking, change her diet and exercise more. She is overextended with family responsibilities, and does not have time to exercise. Her only reprieve is food and an occasional smoke on the back porch. Melina knows she is stressed. She was hoping that her HCP would "read between the lines," validate her depression, and refer her to a counselor.

She has tried the recommended herbs, massage and prayer. They have been minimally helpful. Other folk treatment remedies she may try include using homeopathic herbs, teas and ointments as well as requesting a spiritual intervention by her Orthodox priest. Teas are used to treat gastrointestinal distress, abdominal pain and upper respiratory infection. In addition, moxibustion, or cupping can be used for more significant illness and also for backaches. Melina hasn't tried that yet. K*ofte,* is a Greek form of cupping in which a cut in the shape of a cross is made on the skin prior to placement of the heated cup. The heated cup then draws the blood up into the glass. It is thought that this improves circulation and removes causative effect of the pain or stress.[71]

Family members are expected to be present if the illness is serious and hospitalization required. Their responsibility is not only to provide support, comfort, and assurance, but to participate in the care as well. In some situations they may want to shield the patient from knowing the diagnosis, even though the patient has not stated this request.

> *Reflective exercise: Caring for the Care Giver*
> 1. *Have you been in Melina's position?*
> 2. *Would you address her physical symptoms first or guide the conversation from the perspective of her stress and exhaustion?*
> 3. *Which Greek values could encourage Melina to care for herself?*
> 4. *What support groups for care givers are available within her community and church? In your institution?*
> 5. *How would you follow up?*

Religion

Along with health practices, religious rituals are considered part of the healing process. Strength and health can be attributed to one's faith and to God's protectiveness. The Greek Orthodox church, based strongly on Holy Scripture, values and relies on the writings of the Church Fathers, the Canons, religious rituals, and the power of the holy spirit. It is through these tenets and rituals that members find their connection to the divine and the sacred powers of healing. Icons, depictions of holy men and women, have sacred significance and serve to connect the individual to the spirit world. Every saint has a purpose, whether it is to heal physically, mentally or to mitigate some social issue. Church members may have altars in their home to display the sacred icons, prayer cards and blessed candles. Daily rituals such as lighting the candle, kissing the icon, and making the sign of the cross ensures safety and protection. It is believed that this day-to-day ritual leads to conversations between parents and children about faith and religious beliefs. Attendance at mass, participation in religious education, and parish social events promote a sense of well being and community.

There is a strong belief in miracles and the power of the saints to be the intercession for life's stressors. Similar to other religious traditions, petitions to the saints or the divine usually include promises of better behavior, forgiveness toward one another, and reaching out to the impoverished of the community. Moreover, an ill person may place an icon, the statue of a saint, or the picture of the Virgin Mary next to their bed at home or in the hospital. Each serves to maintain a healing connection with the divine with the hope of a miraculous recovery. Other strategies include purification rituals, seeking counsel from the priest, as well as congregational support. The priest may use holy oils to draw a cross on the site of the body to be healed. Holy water may act as a healer of body and soul and to cleanse the individual of sin. Perhaps both Theodora and Melina are considering these options as well.

Summary

Unaccustomed to living in this new country, coupled with intergenerational issues, is an everyday challenge for Theodora. Even though she lives with her daughter's family, she continues to feel a sense of isolation and unfamiliarity. For Melina, taking care of her mother and finding time to care for herself is overwhelming. Both mother and daughter voice multiple somatic ailments that perhaps, reflect inner uncertainty. As HCPs we need to understand the cultural influence on decisions and actions surrounding healthcare.

Culture Care Decisions & Actions

Acknowledge & Affirm
Focus on the family, not individual
Work with delegated family leader
Maintain hospitality
Participate in church activities

Discuss & Adjust
Identify Greek community resources
Empathetic listening - don't force disclosure
Allow time (coffee/chitchat)
Encourage visit with priest.

Collaborate & Change
Nutrition review
Exercise regime
Encourage time for self care

The Caregiver Assessment Grid was developed by *The Michigan Dementia Coalition*. The following list offers assessments tools that measure quality of life, memory, caregiver burden among other items. They are available to the public.

- The Zarit Burden Interview
    - 12 item assessment
    - Examines subjective burden, financial & emotional burden and more

- The Pearling Caregiver Stress Scales
    - 15 item assessment focus on cognitive states
    - "Yes" answers link to supportive websites

- The Risk Appraisal Measure (RAM)
    - 16 item assessment - usually takes 5-7 minutes
    - Examines six domains of caregiver risk

- The Geriatric Depression Scale
    - Two versions - 30 question & 15 question
    - Yes & No answers

- The Caregiver Burden Scale
    - Adapted from the Family Practice Notebook
    - 22 item version

- The Center for Epidemiology Studies Depression Scale
    - 20 item self report
    - Measures depressive feelings & behaviors for past week

Resources

Archakis, A., Papazachariou, D. (2008). Prosodic cues of identity construction: Intensity in Greek young women's conversational narratives. *Journal of Sociolinguistics.* 12(5): 627-647.

Athanasiou, A., Papathanassoglou, E.D., Patiraki, E., McCarthy, M.S., Giannakopoulou, M. (2014). Family visitation in Greek intensive care units: Nurses' perspective. *American Journal of Critical Care.* 23(4): 326-333.

Billis, E., McCarthy, C.J., Gliatis, J., Stathopoulos, I., Papandreou, M., Oldham, J.A. (2010). Which are the most important discriminatory items for sub classifying non-specific low back pain? A Delphi study among Greek health professionals. *Journal of Evaluation in Clinical Practice.* 16: 542-549.

Crea, T.M. (2012). Faith practices and life stress: An exploratory study of parishioners within the Greek Orthodox Archdiocese of American. *Journal of Psychology and Christianity.* 31(3): 227-241.

Fouka, G., Plakas, S., Taket, A., Boudioni, M., Dandoulakis, M. (2012). Health-related religious rituals of the Greek Orthodox church: Their uptake and meanings. *Journal of Nursing Management.* 20:1058-1068.

Francis, A., Papageorgiou, P. (2004). Expressed emotion in Greek versus Anglo-Saxon families of individuals with schizophrenia. *Australian Psychologist.* 39(2): 172-177.

Galanis, P., Sourtzi, P., Bellali, T., Theodorou, M., Karamitri, I., Siskou, O., Charalambous, G., Kaitelidou, D. Public health services knowledge and utilization among immigrants in Greece: A cross-sectional study. *BMC Health Services Research.* 13:350-358.

Higginbottom, F., Richter, M.S., Young, S., Ortiz, L.M., Callender, S.D., Forgeron, J.I., Boyce, M.L. (2012). Evaluating the utility of the FamCHAT ethnocultural nursing assessment tool at a Canadian tertiary care hospital: A pilot study with recommendation for hospital management. *Journal of Nursing Education and Practice.* 2(2): 24-40.

Hurley, C., Panagiotopoulos, G., Tsianikas, M., Newman, L., Walker, R. (2013). Access and acceptability of community-based services for older Greek migrants in Australia: User and provider perspectives. *Health and Social Care in the Community.* 21(2): 140-149.

Hyphantis, T., Kroenke, K., Papatheodorou, E., Paika, V., Theocharopoulos, N., Ninou, A., Tomenson, B., Carvalho, A.F., Guthrie, E. Validity of the Greek version of the PHQ 15-item somatic symptom severity scale in patients with chronic medical conditions and correlations with emergency department use and illness perceptions. *Comprehensive Psychiatry.* 55: 1950-1959.

Issari, P. (2011). Greek American ethnic identity, cultural experience and the 'embodied language' of dance: Implication for counseling. *International Journal of Advanced Counseling.* 33: 252-265.

Jurgens, J. Greek American. *Countries and their cultures.* Retrieved June 17, 2016 from www.everyculture.com/multi/Du-Ha/Greek-American.

Killian, K.D., Agathangelou, A.M. (2005). Greek Families. In M. McGoldrick, Giordano, J., Garcia-Preto, N. (Eds.) Ethnicity & Family Therapy. (3rd Ed.). New York: The Guilford Press.

Langman, N. (2016). Caregivers of dementia patients: Mental health screening & support. *Clinical Reviews.* 26(6): 42-50.

Michigan Dementia Coalition. Caregiver Assessment Tool Grid. The Rosalynn Carter Ins.www.rosalynncarter.org/UserFiles/Michigan%20Assessment%20Grid.pdf Accessed September 30, 2016.

Mitchison, D., Sze, M., Butow, P., Aldridge, L., Hui, R., Vardy, J., Eisenbrunch, M., Iedema, R., Goldstein, D. (2012). Prognostic communication preferences of migrant patients and their relatives. *Psycho-Oncology.* 21: 496-504.

Moisoglou, I., Panagiotis, P., Galanis, P., Siskou, O., Maniadakis, N., Kaitelidou, D. (2014).Conflict management in a Greek public hospital: Collaboration or avoidance. *International Journal of Caring Sciences.* 7(1). 75-82.

Mystakidou, K., Tsilika, E., Parpa, E., Katsouda, E., Vlahos, L. (2003). A Greek perspective on concepts of death and expression of grief, with implications for practice. *International Journal of Palliative Nursing.* 9(12): 534-537.

Nishimura, S., Nevgi, A., Tella, S. (2009). Communication style and cultural features in high/low context communication cultures: A case study of Finland, Japan and India. 783-796.

Papadopoulos, I. (1999). Health and illness beliefs of Greek Cypriots living in London. *Journal of Advanced Nursing.* 29(5): 1097-1104.

Portes, A., Zhou, M. (1993). The new second generation: Segmented assimilation and its variants. American Academy of Political and Social Science 530(1), 74-96.

Purnell, L.D., Paulanka, B.J. (2005). People of Greek Heritage. *Guide to Culturally Competent Health Care.* Pennsylvania: F.A.Davis Company.

Rosenbaum, J.N. (1991). The health meanings and practices of older Greek-Canadian widows. *Journal of Advanced Nursing.* 16: 1320-1327.

Conchita's Story
There is no such thing as too much weight.. | 17

Obesity - Cuban Family

"It wasn't so long ago," Conchita mused, " that whistles would surround me as I bicycled through the streets of Havana. My senos almost hit the handlebars and when I went over a bump, dios mio, they bounced like flan. It did get to the point when my nalda extended a little too far beyond that puny seat they put on all the bikes you could find there that I gave up riding. But no one complained there that I was too fat. There was no such thing."

Cobchita's shortness of breath, once attractive and sexy, is getting to be a little scary. Her sons Miguelito and Jorge are worried for their mother. They try their best not to resemble her too much, though ---some of their classmates call her "Conchita Chito"---and it is hard to keep from sampling the old country food when the extended family celebrates fiestas de los santos. They are both good at sports, thankfully. Miguelito is a wrestler and needs to keep his weight down to *qualify, and Jorge wins medals at track. Even though they love her dearly, they are still a little embarrassed by their mother. And worried.*

Conchita is sitting in the waiting room of Clinica Ole. It has been difficult for her to get into the tiny chair in the first place, but at least it has no arms trying to hold her in; when there are arms it's a struggle getting onto the seat and even worse attempting to extricate herself. First, squeak. Then, pop. The employment office has those nasty chairs with arms. The receptionist there wasn't simpatica anyway, couldn't even speak Spanish. Conchita had seen her expression when she walked in:

"Oh, here we go. Another Big Mama looking for a job, as if she could find a spot that would accommodate such a strain on company health benefits..."

"Why did I let Tia Blanca convince me to leave mi patria? She kept talking about the Communidad here, all those Cubans who'd fled back in the 50's, but when I snuck into Florida with mis hijos all I saw beyond my family were snooty Gringo-types, the skinny light-skinned patrons who'd owned the farms. Doesn't mi tia remember that we worked for those folk? They don't go to Clinica Ole, much less a curandera. No herbs for them except ginger ale and gin!"

Reflective exercise: Obesity, Culture & Health
1. *Do you or someone in your family struggle with weight?*
2. *Is being overweight seen as a sign of health and prosperity in your cultural group?*
3. *Do you think the concerns of Conchita's sons will influence her to change her eating regime?*
4. *How would you respond if she said she "likes being overweight" and does not see there is a problem?*
5. *If she does not acknowledge the potential health concerns, what is your next step?*

Obesity in America

Being overweight, in some cultures and ethnic groups, is viewed as "healthy." In others, it is seen as glutinous and unhealthy – people who cannot control their dietary intake. Many overweight persons face prejudice and discrimination in the work place and also within their family. Conchita's children are concerned about her health and a possible future without her in their lives. They are embarrassed about her size, too.

The Hispanic Health and Nutrition Examination (HHANE) survey indicates that 34% of Cuban American females are overweight. This compares with 25% of Puerto Rican women and 30% of Mexican women.[72] Obesity, in the United States, has received a great deal of attention in the past several years, due to the direct correlation with heart disease, diabetes, cancer and osteoarthritis. According to the Department of Health and Human Services, the prevalence of obesity in adults living in the United States has increased from 13.4% in 1960 to 35.7% today. Current numbers issued by the Center for Disease Control indicate that the obesity rate ranges from a low of 9% in Asians, to a high of 51% for Blacks. In 2012, more than one third of children and adolescents were overweight or obese. [73]

How did we get so obese over the past 50 years? The most significant factor was a shift from daily physical activity to a sedentary lifestyle. Furthermore, the development and consumption of processed foods and soft drinks have added more salt, fat and sugar to our daily dietary intake. While these are just a few of the culprits, others factors, such as extended work hours, lead to fast food purchases and poor nutritional choices. The change in lifestyle and eating habits have resulted in the gradual, but steady, increase in weight and body mass index (BMI).

How does one determine if they are a normal weight, overweight or obese? Calculating the BMI is the answer. A ratio of height to weight determines the BMI. The normal range is 18.5 to 24.9; overweight is 25-29.9; and obese is 30+ (Figure 15-1).[74] BMI findings, waist circumference, along with risk factors such as high triglycerides, blood sugar, high cholesterol, and high blood pressure are definitive predictors of heart disease and diabetes. Review the chart below – where do you find yourself?

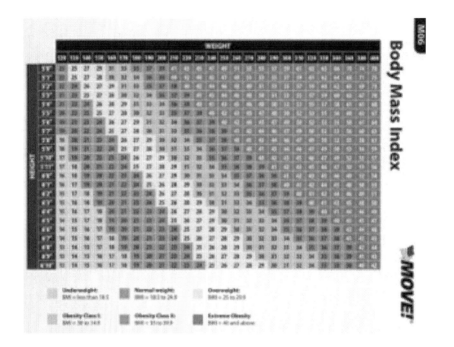

Figure 15-1 Body Mass Index

In response to the obesity epidemic in children, Michelle Obama, America's First Lady, initiated the *Let's Move* program in 2010. While directed at obesity in children and adolescents, this informative and interactive message became relevant to adults as well. Perhaps it is time for healthcare providers to "get on board" and not only address this problem with our patients, but also confront our own weight issues.

Conchita did not begin her life overweight. However, in the Cuban culture, being overweight is viewed as attractive and a sign of good health – especially in children and women. She acknowledges her large size, but does not seem motivated to change her life style or dietary intake. However, her sons are important to her, thus perhaps inviting them into the conversation at her next appointment may serve as a catalyst to change her eating habits that began in childhood.

History

Cuba was under the occupation of Spain for more than three hundred years. Emancipation was the outcome of the Spanish American War of 1898. The United States became an overseer. The Platt Amendment, written into the Cuban constitution, gave the United States the right to intervene in Cuban affairs as needed. U.S. peace keeping troops remained a presence on the island until 1934. Following the change in regimes, many Cubans emigrated to Florida and New York. They primarily worked in the tobacco fields. In contrast to the Mexican migrant experience, these laborers were accompanied by their families, thus communities formed and people stayed. Cuba remained bound to the United States until the revolution in 1959 when Fidel Castro took control from President Fulgencia Batista. He established a socialist state. Life changed dramatically for those residents in the middle and upper class.

Between 1959 and 1965 there were four waves of immigrants to the United States. This was in direct response to social and political change. Those who had supported Castro in the revolution, left because of failed promises by his regime and the threat of communist rule. Others were business people, large land owners and supporters of Batista. It is thought that over 700,000 persons left Cuba during that time. Due to this large and sudden influx of refugees, President John F. Kennedy signed the Migration and Refugee Assistance Act of 1962 which assured financial appropriations to provide services to refugees. An office was established in Miami to deal with the nearly two thousand people arriving each week. Assistance included financial aid, educational loans, healthcare, adult education and re-training, resettlement and care of unaccompanied children.

In the years to follow more diverse groups of immigrants arrived. In 1963, following the Bay of Pigs event, prisoners, released by Castro, were encouraged to emigrate to the United States. In 1965 he opened the Port of Camarioca, allowing Cuban exiles to return to the island for the sole purpose of evacuating their relatives. It came with a price – those leaving had to forfeit their land and property. The final wave came in 1980 with the Marielitos. They were named for the Cuban port of Mariel and were mainly working class and unemployed people. Their boats were generally overcrowded and barely seaworthy. Many lost their lives.

Today Cubans make up about four percent of the Hispanic population in the United States and experience a higher socioeconomic status and educational level than their forerunners. Cubans radiate vibrant and economically stable communities in which family, heritage and history play a vital role.

Cultural Beliefs & Values

The most important value for refugees was pride in their Cuban culture and heritage. Today, many continue to have a passionate connection with the past, even though embracing a strong identity with being an American. Recently during a Cultural Awareness seminar in Florida, a participant shared his story with me. At age six, he left Cuba with his family. While many decades have passed, and he has done well in this country, he said he recently became nostalgic for his roots. "I can still remember the house and street we lived on. For some reason it is important, for me, to go back and visit the place I called "home," even if it was for only six years. It is a piece of me." American literary critic Gustavo Pérez-Firmat would call him a "one-and-a-half" – children born in Cuba and growing up in the United States. The story of the Cuban American family experience must be told as an intergenerational narrative of love, loyalty and longing.[75] Therefore, many choose to live in a community that preserves their language and promotes their values and beliefs. Family loyalty and obligation are strong values held by Cuban Americans. Extended family, grandparents, aunts, uncles, those related by blood and those not (friends) play a significant role in this structure. Collectivist in nature, all are a source of support emotionally, physically and financially.

Cultural Beliefs & Values

Familismo
Pride in Culture & Heritage
Collectivistic - Interdependence
Simpatico & Personalismo
Religion & Spirituality

> *Reflective exercise: Culture & Health*
> 1. *Which cultural values would you incorporate into your discussion with Conchita about her obesity?*
> 2. *Are there other family members to include in this conversation?*
> 3. *Are your cultural values and beliefs the same or different?*
> 4. *Now that you've discovered "common ground" which value do you think would be most effective to encourage her to rethink being overweight is "fine with her."*

Communication

The core values of effective communication within the Cuban culture is simpatica and personalismo. Both highlight the importance of respect and courtesy, which ensures smooth and personal relationships. Avoidance of conflict or harsh criticism are reflective of this value. While Cuban Americans may appear loud and aggressive to outsiders, this is considered normal within the community. Furthermore, being animated, along with frequent interruptions, is expected. Hand gestures add to and reinforce the message. Eye contact, an important aspect especially in formal situations, indicates that one is engaged in the conversation. Absence of eye contact could be interpreted as insincerity or disrespect. Choteo, a form of humor, is displayed as ridiculing one another or exaggerating something out of proportion. It serves to reduce tension, especially during social encounters. It is said to promote interpersonal closeness with family and friends.

According to the US Census, 83% of Cubans speak a language other than English at home. While first generation speak primarily Spanish, second and third generation are more likely bilingual. Many elderly prefer to have their adult children translate for them. This conflicts with the law which states that a family member can translate only in the case of emergency. Therefore, it is important to share the hospital/clinic policy regarding translators and then give them an option by asking the question – "Some people prefer using a translator, others prefer a family member – which do you prefer?" It is important for the patient to understand the HCP's responsibility to protect their privacy. Yet, it is in offering options that they recognize their right to decide.

> *Reflective exercise: Communication*
> 1. *How would you demonstrate personalism & simpatico in the conversation?*
> 2. *Are you comfortable with Conchita's expressive and loud style?*
> 3. *Recognizing humor is used to exaggerate, how would you accurately evaluate her dietary intake or exercise regime?*

Time Orientation

Culture places varying levels of importance on time. Cubans have a more casual approach which translates into possibly arriving late for an appointment. This view is changing with acculturation. While the elderly are present and/or past oriented, second and third generations adhere to a more punctual schedule, along with a focus on future educational achievements and economical aspirations.

For some newly arrived immigrants, or the elderly, their thought is that "one day I'll return to Cuba." The gentleman from the conference, now 58 years old, talked about returning to see his "homeland." It is vital to understand that the past still is an integral part of the Cuban narrative. Listening to their story and understanding the values placed on their culture and family are vital aspects to consider during interactions.

Familioso . . . Family

Inclusion of the extended family is expected for Cuban Americans. This may include Compadres (godparents), aunts, uncles, cousins and more. The values of personalismo and respect are integral to these family dynamics. Familioso, connotes a loyalty and responsibility to family members. It is the core value of their identity and provides an assurance of emotional, physical and financial support. Family needs are considered more important than an individual member's needs. As a result, tension occurs with succeeding generations who are trying to balance the collectivistic Cuban and the individualistic American values.

Adolescents, trying to find their identity by the rejection of Cuban values, traditions and heritage may seem disrespectful to their parents and grandparents. Obligation to family is an additional source of tension for the young adult who wants to attend college away from home or seek employment out of state. As a result, this creates a division that seems insurmountable. Parents cannot understand why their son/daughter can't just "move back home" and live next door. The young adult children want to "see the world" first and then decide the next step.

It is common to have several generations living within a household or next door. Families are generally hierarchal with the father as the head of the household. With acculturation, this is changing. As more women are entering the workforce and contributing financially to the family, it is not uncommon to hear about men who are assuming some household responsibilities. Yet, traditional ways are still relevant. Generally, the father is responsible for financial stability and seen as protector. The mother's responsibility is child care, home maintenance, health concerns, and providing the emotional support for the family members.

Children are highly valued and pampered. They are taught to be respectful of their parents and elders, and expected to live at home until marriage. They maintain a strong relationship with their parents throughout their life. Grandparents are given respect not only by their children and grandchildren, but also the Cuban community. They are a integral part of the family. They provide child care and offer insights into health decisions and actions. It is important to ask the patient, "How are decisions made in your family?" This provides an insight for the HCP to fully understand the family structure and dynamics.

Religion

Considering Cuba's history of occupation by Spain, it is not surprising that the majority of Cuban Americans are Roman Catholic. Many believe in a strong personal relationship with the Virgin Mary, Jesus, and the saints who act as their emissaries to God. In addition, Catholic priests provide healing sacraments and prayers especially during times of illness and uncertainty. Crucifixes, portraits and statues of the Virgin Mary, Jesus and the saints may be displayed at the entrance to the home or business. There may be an altar or shrine inside the home as well. A family member may place a photo of a saint on the ill person's pillow. This is thought to provide comfort and reassurance that health will return.

In addition, some Cuban Americans ascribe to and integrate elements of the Yoruba tribal beliefs brought by slaves from Nigeria to Cuba. These slaves were forced to be baptized into Roman Catholicism. However, many kept their own beliefs. Santeria, a religious/spiritual practice, includes both Yoruba and Catholic beliefs. They worship African gods called *orishas* and perform healing rituals such as animal sacrifice and magic to thwart spirit possession. Santeros, those trained in the practice of Santeria, are consulted in cases of soul loss, illness and intrusion by an evil spirit. Both *orishas* and *saints* are acknowledged and worshipped for their protection and healing powers.

Health Practices

Cuban Americans ascribe to biomedicine and traditional healing practices. Family is the primary source for all health information and counsel. Santero's counsel is sought for physical healing along with insights to the emotional or spiritual component of the illness. They use medicinal properties of plants, herbs, stones and charms to restore health and provide protection. Moreover, they act as an intercessory between the real and spirit world to cure and to ease pain. Botanicas, operated by Santeros, specialize in herbs, potions, religious articles, and other healing remedies. These stores are frequented by many Cuban Americans who seek a cure, want to ward off an evil spirit, or need to break a curse. The use of complementary mind-body practices, religious rituals, and herbal remedies usually precede an appointment with the HCP. A person may wait until the illness is viewed as a crisis before making an appointment.

The role of the sick person and that of family members is very clear. It is culturally acceptable for the ill person to be passive and totally dependent on others during illness. Expressions of pain and discomfort are expected. It is believed that these expression will cause the pain to subside. If hospitalized, there is an expectations of visitors, gifts, cards and flowers. During this time, extended family helps with household responsibilities such as meal preparation and child care. The community is a source of support during these times of illness and uncertainty.

> *Reflective exercise: Some questions for Conchita*
> 1. *In American culture, thin is considered attractive and healthy which is contrary to Conchita's belief ~ where can you find common ground?*
> 2. *What Cuban foods does she enjoy? Are there low fat recipes she can use to make Cuban dishes?*
> 3. *In addition to her biking, what other activities does she enjoy?*

Summary

Obesity, in many cultures, is not thought of as an illness. This is a dilemma for the HCP. Acknowledging the direct correlation between obesity and heart disease, diabetes and cancer, how do we convey this information to Conchita in a respectful and culturally sensitive manner? First, we acknowledge that obesity is considered healthy by her culture. Next, we can ask her – "From your perspective, what are the consequences of obesity?" Perhaps this leads to a discussion of the Cuban American cultural value of loyalty to her children and her parents. It may be helpful to include her sons at the appointment to share their concerns. Creating an awareness that health issues related to obesity may eventually impact her ability to be with her family could be the impetus for change.

Acknowledging that food and socialization are integral to the Cuban American lifestyle, discussion of her dietary intake is essential. Perhaps the HCP could begin by asking her to identify Cuban foods that she considers fresh and healthy. This provides the segues into a discussion about how those foods are rich in vitamins, minerals, protein and carbohydrate and lower in calories. The message is clear – it's not about taking food away, rather providing familiar food in a new venue.

Lastly, exercise – something few people *want* to do. Yet, let's look at it with new eyes. Perhaps a Zumba class with Cuban music (rich in heritage and past), a Sunday walk following church or a bike ride with her sons would be enjoyable. Involving family in the discussion assures a greater likelihood of success and good health. Working collaboratively demonstrates respect for culture and a willingness to incorporate new concepts that lead to healthy outcomes.

Culture Care Decisions and Actions

Acknowledge & Affirm
Family involvement - specifically her sons
Extended family assistance
Cuban heritage and past

Discuss & Adjust
Decrease fat intake
Keep a food & exercise diary

Collaborate & Change
Encourage Diverse Exercise - Dancing & Walking
Increase vegetables, lean meats & fruit

Resources

Alcántara, C., Chen, C.N., Alegría, M. (2014). Transnational ties and past-year major depressive episodes among Latino immigrants. *Cultural Diversity and Ethnic Minority Psychology.* pp. 1-10. http://dx.doi.org/10.1037/a0037540

Bernal, G., Shapiro, E. (2005). Cuban Families. In McGoldrick, M.M. *Ethnicity & Family Therapy.* (3rd Ed.). New York: The Guilford Press.

Diaz, M.E., Jiménez, S., Garcia, R.G., Bonet, M., Wong, I. (2009). Overweight, obesity, central adiposity and associated chronic diseases in Cuban adults. *MEDICC Review.* 11(4). pp. 23-28.

Exebio, J.C., Zarini, G.G., Exebio, C., Huffman, F. (2011). Healthy eating index scores associated with symptoms of depression in Cuban-Americans with and without type 2 diabetes: A cross sectional study. *Nutrition Journal.* 10:135-142.

Franco, M.A., Wilson, T. (2013). Cuban Americans. In Giger, J.N. (Ed.). *Transcultural Nursing: Assessment & Intervention.* (6th Ed.).

Friedemann, M.L., Buckwalter, K.C., Newman, F.L., Mauro, A.C. (2013). Patterns of Caregiving of Cuban, other Hispanic Caribbean Black, and White elders in South Florida. *Journal of Cross Cultural Gerontology.* 28:137-152.

Huffman, F.G., Vaccaro, J.A., Gundupalli, D., Zarini, G.G., Dixon, Z. (2012). Acculturation and diabetes self-management of Cuban Americans: Is age a protective factor? *Ageing International.* 37:195-209.

Khan, L.K., Sobal, J., Martorell, R. (1997) Acculturation, socioeconomic status and obesity in Mexican Americans, Cuban Americans, and Puerto Ricans. *International Journal of Obesity.* 21:91-96.

Marks, G., Garcia, M. Solis, J.M. (1990). Health risk behaviors of Hispanics in the United States: Findings from HHANES, 1982-84. *American Journal of Public Health.* 80:20-26.

Morales, L.S., Lara, M., Kington, R.S., Valdez, R.O., Escarce, J.J. (2002). Socioeconomic cultural and behavioral factors affecting Hispanic health outcomes. *Journal of Health Care for the Poor and the Underserved.*

13(4). 477-503.
National Institute of Health. (2013). We Can. www.nhibi.nih.gove/health/eduational/we can.
Ogden, C.L., Carroll, M.D., Kit, B.K., Flegal, K.M. (2013). Prevalence of obesity among adults: United States, 2011-2012. National Center for Health Statistics. NCHS Data Brief. No. 131.(2012).
Pena, M.S., Patel, D., Leyva, D.R., Khan, B.V., Sperling, L. (2012). Lifestyle risk factors and cardiovascular disease in Cubans and Cuban Americans. *Cardiology Research and Practice.* 2012: 1-6.
Pulgarón, E.R., Patiño-Fernández, A.M., Sanchez, J., Carrillo, A., Delamater, A.M. (2013). Hispanic children and the obesity epidemic: Exploring the role of abuelas. *Family Systems and Health.* 31(3). 274-279.
Purnell, L. D., Gil, J. (2013). People of Cuban Heritage. In Purnell, L.D. (Ed.) *Transcultural Health Care: A Culturally competent approach.* (4th Ed.) PA: F.A. Davis.
Solis, J.M., Marks, G., Garcia, M., Shelton, D. (1990). Acculturation, access to care and use of preventive service by Hispanics: Findings from HHANES 1982-84. *American Journal of Public Health.* 80:11-19.
Torres, J.M., Wallace, S.P. (2014). Migration circumstances, psychological distress, and self-rated physical health for Latino immigrants in the United States. *Research and Practice.* 103(9). 1619-1627.
U.S. Department of Commerce, Bureau of the Census. (2011). *This Hispanic Population: 2010.* Washington D.C.: U.S. Government Printing Office.
U.S. Department of Commerce, Bureau of the Census. (2009). *American Community Survey, Cubans.* Washington D.D.: U.S. Government Printing Office.
U.S. Department of Health and Human Services. Wasem, R.E. (2009). Cuban migration to the United States: Policy and Trends. *Congressional Research Service.* pp.1-20. Retrieved on May 6, 2015 from www.crs.gov.
U.S. Department of Health and Human Services. (2012). Overweight and obesity statistics. National Institute of Health. NIH Publication No. 04-4158.

Carlito's Story

I Can't Breath! | 18

Asthma - Prison - Puerto Rican Family

    Carlito shakes his head to get the dust from his nose. He lies in the dirt in A yard, one of many inmates caught outside when the alarm sounded; they are all required to lie face down until a guard OKs movement. Carlito coughs hard, trying to breathe. These codes still catch him off guard even after a year of incarceration. Asthma was hard enough on the streets of New Jersey, but there he had an inhaler when he could afford one, and amazingly the stresses of poverty and injustice he faced daily did not seem as brutal as they do "inside." He had his family in Trenton plus those back in Puerto Rico, and he knew they all prayed for him. He was trusted and respected by his homies. He was a team player. Here he misses his mother and his auntie *every day, especially when he thinks of how they used to visit each weekend when he was in the Mercer County Jail.*

In prison, he is an "other." Neither the Nortenos nor the Surenos accept him entirely, since their own shared language doesn't seem to let them mix despite the reality that they're from the same country originally. Incredible. Here there are at least two distinct Mexican groups, plus blacks, AMIs [Native Americans], whites, and "others." Carlito's best buddies are men from Guam and the Philippines, interestingly. They are "others" too. Of course sometimes he just nods when they comment appreciatively on a particular TV show that he doesn't like much, but friends are vital in here.

Carlito is getting scared. His lungs are aching as he tries to breathe. The dirt keeps getting into his mouth or is it his nose? These attacks really are attacking him; they're almost as bad as that first one he remembers when he started Woodrow Wilson Elementary.

"I bet the C.O.s won't believe me in the midst of a code when I say I can't get my breath. Seem to be only the tough ones out here right now too. I sure wish Dr. Satay would poke his head out of the clinic. Don't panic, Carlito. Don't panic."

Life and Health in the Prison

"Before entering prison, approximately one in seven inmates was taking a prescription medication for an active medical problem. However, upon incarceration 20.9% of federal, 24.3% of State and 36.5% of local-jail inmates stopped their medication."

Andrew Wilper MD 2009

> *Reflective exercise: Your views . . . .*
> 1. *Have you or someone you know spent time in prison?*
> 2. *Do you believe prisoners should receive the health care comparable to services received in the community?*
> 3. *If not, why not?*
> 4. *If a prison offered care equal to the local community – do you think it would promote a more healthy lifestyle once released?*

Currently . . .

. . . there are more than 2.2 million adults confined to state and federal prisons, and county jails. The United States incarcerates more people per capita, approximately 800 per 100,000, than any other country. Men make up the majority of the prison population. Blacks comprise the greater part of inmates (37%), followed by whites (32%) and Hispanics (22%) with "other" (Asian, Native American, Alaskan Native) comprising the remaining 8%. The majority have not completed high school. While the predominant age of the prisoners is less than 39 years old, more than 33% – an 8% increase over the past 10 years – are older than 50.[76] Consequently, chronic health conditions are more prevalent and require increased funding for healthcare services.

In the past, healthcare was not readily available to prisoners. That was until 1976 when a case, citing lack of quality healthcare, was brought before the Supreme Court – Estelle v Gamble. Citing the Eighth Amendment, the plaintiff, an inmate in a state prison, claimed he was subjected to cruel and unusual punishment because he did not receive adequate treatment for a back injury incurred while doing prison work. The Supreme Court ruled in favor of the plaintiff and established that states must provide healthcare that meets community standards. Following this ruling, the American Medical Association received a grant from the Law Enforcement Alliance of American to establish medical standards of care for prisons. The project was entitled "Healthcare in Correctional Institutions." These standards continue to be revised and updated.

Unfortunately, many who enter prison today do not receive adequate healthcare. The percentage of inmates with diabetes, hypertension, mental illness, and asthma is higher than the general population. "Among inmates with a persistent medical problem, 13.9% of federal inmates, 20.1% of state inmates and 68.4% of local jail inmates had received no medical examination . . . and those with active medical problems for which laboratory monitoring is routinely indicated had not undergone at least one blood test since incarceration."[77] Furthermore, The Pew Report in 2012 stated that Hepatitis C, found in 25-40% of the prison population, accounts for upward of $30,000 per inmate. [78] There are those who believe that taxpayer's money should not be spent on prisoners. Yet, from a humanistic standpoint, and as mandated by the Supreme Court, inmates are entitled to healthcare. Our scenario highlights just such an incident. Carlito, a twenty-six year old Puerto Rican, with a long history of asthma, has not received adequate care. Research shows that Puerto Ricans have the highest rate of asthma of all ethnic groups – higher than non Hispanic whites, black and all other Hispanic subgroups. They are three times more likely to use Emergency services to restore health. [79]

The Puerto Rican story

Puerto Rico, a small island in the Northeast part of the Caribbean, was once the home of the Taino Indians. They called their island Borinquen. Life changed with the arrival of Christopher Columbus in 1493. He claimed the island for Spain. Tobacco, sugarcane and coffee plantations followed. The Taino Indians, and those brought from Africa, worked as slaves on these estates. Many died from starvation, disease, and overwork. Following the Spanish American War of 1898, Puerto Rico was ceded to the United States and became a Territory. The United States then created a civil government, made leadership appointments, and retained the right to veto any laws proposed. A representative of Puerto Rico, similar to the delegate from Washington DC, was given a seat in the U.S. House of Representative. However the delegate did not have voting privileges.

The transitional years were arduous. It was difficult to adapt to the requirements established by the United States. In 1917 residents were granted U.S. Citizenship, thus they could travel between Puerto Rico and the United

Sates freely. Puerto Ricans made two bids at independence, once in 1950 and again in 1954. Following those failed attempts, emigration to the U.S. began in earnest. Puerto Ricans, similar to other immigrant groups, were seeking employment, education, and a better life for their families. It was at this time that Carlito's grandparents came to New York City.

Puerto Ricans living in the United States, continue to have a strong sense of nationality and loyalty to their home country. They self-identify as Puerto Rican, Puertorriqueños or Baricus, the Taino Indian word for Puerto Rican. According to the U.S. Census Bureau, they are the second largest Hispanic subgroup in the United States, comprising approximately 9% of the population. Most were born in the United States and reside primarily in the Northeast (53%) and South (30%). However, cities such as Chicago boast of the second largest Puerto Rican population (177,000) in the country, followed by Los Angeles (48,000). Although they have the second highest educational attainment within the Hispanic group, poverty abounds at 28%.[80] While those living at or below the poverty level qualify for financial assistance to purchase health insurance, the cost of drugs and treatment are prohibitive, as noted in Carlito's story. As a result, families come together to provide the financial support to ensure that care is received.

Cultural Beliefs & Values

Reminiscent of the Taino way of life, Puerto Ricans maintain a peaceful demeanor. A sense of place and family along with the interconnectedness of community is highly valued. It is from this context that we juxtapose the key elements of Carlito's Puerto Rican cultural beliefs, values and health practices with the culture of prison. Where do we find common ground? Each play an integral role in providing healthcare. From our narrative, we know that Carlito has been in prison for more than three years. Always in his thoughts is earning an early parole and reuniting with his family and community.

In the Puerto Rican culture, respect and loyalty are significant values. Respect acknowledges the social worthiness of each person. It is especially important when addressing and interacting with elders, adults and those in authority. Loyalty to family assures protection and care for life. Interdependence, sharing what one has with another, provides assurance of stability within the family structure as well as financial, emotional, and physical support.

Many of these values are present in the prison setting as well. Loyalty to, and sharing with other inmates within the confines of the prison assures camaraderie and security. Likewise, those same values are relevant to health and prison staff as well. Collaboration, coordination and cooperation with colleagues maintains security and safety. However, cultural beliefs, values and health practices of inmates and healthcare staff may conflict, thus lead to misunderstanding and mistrust. Acknowledgement by prison staff of cultural differences improves communication and facilitates and understanding of decisions and actions of all involved. As you review the beliefs and values listed, reflect on your beliefs and values and ask yourself "If I were a prison guard or a healthcare staff where would I find common ground with Carlito?"

Cultural Beliefs and Values

Dignity, Honor & Respect
Familismo ~ Family First ~ Loyalty to Family
Interdependence ~ Collectivistic ~ Cooperation
Trusting Others
Religion & Spirituality
Personalismo ~ Simpatia

Family ~ Familismo

Family comes first in all circumstances. Carlito's family continues to be supportive and present in his life. They visit regularly, which provides him with the assurance that when paroled, the support and security of a loving family are waiting– unconditionally. Family, in the Puerto Rican culture, extends beyond nuclear to include those related by blood and marriage. Collectivistic in nature, family is considered a network, a kinship which relies on the interdependent approach of mutual obligation.

While the more traditional Puerto Rican family is patriarchal, those acculturated into the mainstream American culture are becoming more egalitarian. Nonetheless, defined gender roles and responsibilities are still evident. The father is considered the head of the household. His responsibility is to provide protection and financial support for the family. Machismo, a term of respect for manliness, exemplifies his ability to fulfill family responsibilities coupled with recognition of his leadership and trustworthiness.

Mothers are held in high esteem throughout their life. The term marianismo, used to describe the mother's attributes, reflects the high regard they have for the Virgin Mary. Mothers are responsible for passing on religious and cultural traditions to their children. In addition to maintaining a home environment, they provide discipline, guidance and counseling. They gain status in the community as they age. Mothers display strength, perseverance, flexibility and the ability to survive regardless of the situation. As a result, we recognize Maria's loyalty to her son that, in spite of the distance she must travel, she visits him monthly.

Children are highly valued, and are the center of family life. Being overweight with rosy red cheeks is thought to be a sign of health and wealth. Raised in a very protective and disciplined environment, children are expected to show respect for parents and elders, and to do well in school. Sons are encouraged to portray a strong and confident demeanor. Daughters are guided to manage home life situations and provide care for their siblings. Both usually live at home until marriage. They are taught at an early age the responsibility to care for their aging parents. Grandparents continue to play an active role in the family, providing child care, teaching traditional values, reinforcing educational activities, and serving as disciplinarians. They are respected by all in the family and the community. Elders usually live with daughters and rarely, if ever, is the decision made to place them in nursing homes.

Family dynamics and culture influence how decisions are made. In the Puerto Rican culture, some families rely on older adults and extended family to participate in that process. The father is the person who conveys the message. Another option is to delegate someone who they believe is more experienced or intelligent, thus ensuring a perceived better outcome. In the prison setting,

Carlito's decisions may come after soliciting input from other inmates, friends and family members.

Communication/Time/Space

While it is customary to learn Spanish before English, more than 80% of Puerto Ricans speak English proficiently. Their communication style is described as peaceful and melodic using hand gestures and facial expressions to augment the message. Feelings and emotions are expressed verbally or through touch. Demonstrating respect is shown using minimal eye contact. Elders are addressed by title – Señor, Señora, Don, Dona, followed by their first name. Children show respect for elders by displaying minimal eye contact and lowering their voice.

Personalismo and *Simpatia* guide all interactions and conversations. *Simpatia* encourages smooth interpersonal relationships, and is shown by politeness and pleasantness. *Personalismo,* is exemplified by maintaining a calm and amiable demeanor. The HCP can display both by a welcoming with a handshake and engaging in a friendly conversation prior to getting to the reason for the appointment. Another important value in the Puerto Rican culture is *saving face.* Disagreeing with an elder or one's HCP, brings shame on oneself and their family. To avoid conflict, the individual may nod in silent agreement thus saving face.

Communication in Prison

HCPs communicate in a linear, concrete, and rational approach, while a Puerto Rican explains his current health condition in an abstract, nonlinear manner. To the HCP is may appear disorderly and chaotic. Asking an inmate "when did these symptoms begin?" may result in a descriptive narrative that highlights multiple incidents in the past before addressing current concerns. Acceptance and respect for an inmates's style of communication is essential to establishing rapport. Primary principle: Listen and validate the concerns presented and reflect back empathy and understanding. A good relationship is the result of time and interest shown in the person's narrative.

There are barriers, though, that challenge that process in prison. From the inmate's viewpoint, the HCP, who works closely with the prison staff, may not be trusted with information about his condition. In addition, the HCP must acknowledge potential biases toward inmates. Disclosing personal information, hugging or touching inmates is taboo. As a result, it may be difficult to demonstrate empathy. However, a display of kindness and respect in this caring versus custody environment, encourages inmates to share their concerns about physical and mental health issues.

> *Reflective exercise: Communication & Culture*
> 1. *How could you incorporate the values of simpatico & personalism into your conversation with Carlito?*
> 2. *Is your communication style linear or abstract – a combination?*
> 3. *Realizing time is limited & you want Carlito to "get to the point" – would you interrupt? Allow him to continue?*
> 4. *Now that you have this information, would you modify your*

Time Orientation – Inside and Outside

Time in the Puerto Rican culture is more social and relaxed than in the mainstream American culture. However, time orientation within the confines of a prison setting is clock oriented and scheduled. Everything is structured throughout the day and night – even the release date. Thinking of leaving prison from Carlito's standpoint is a future aspiration he rarely considers. From his perspective, the past may be viewed as better than the present – "todo tiempo pasado es mejor que el tiempo present" (everything in the past was better than the present). Because he may focus on the time prior to incarceration, he may lack the motivation to engage in a conversation about asthma treatment which could affect future health.

Health Practices

In his youth, Carlito's asthma was exacerbated by poor housing, lack of access to care, and financial constraints. His parents did not have the resources or the time to take him to the neighborhood clinic. He learned to endure the symptoms as long as possible until they became so severe that he needed to go to the emergency room via ambulance. In prison though, waiting until the last minute to call for help, could be life threatening. Unfortunately Carlito is convinced that the health staff see him as a chronic complainer and someone who waits until the last minute to call for assistance. Now more than ever, Carlito's faith and family beliefs are core to maintaining his health and well being. He remembers well his grandmother's stories about why people get sick and why they die. He also knows her deep faith in the ability to heal. When he experienced asthma attacks as a child, he heard her praying to God and the saints, invoking their intervention. Healing always followed.

Causes of illness, according to the Puerto Rican culture, include the imbalance of hot and cold, lack of personal attention to health, breaking commandments, disharmony within one's body, or discord in relationships with family/friends or God. Most Puerto Ricans hold a fatalistic view of life, ascribing to an external locus of control which deems the power of outside forces affect one's health and well-being. Regardless, the belief is that health can be restored by insuring a balance between hot and cold, paying attention to healthy lifestyle, mending relationships and offering penance for breaking commandments.

In addition to the healing rituals offered by a Catholic priest, many Puerto Ricans hold a strong belief in Santeria. Santeria, a magicoreligious practice, is a combination of African and Catholic spiritual beliefs. The Santero, considered a priest and traditional healer, has the ability to identify a person's problem, provide treatment, and counsel them on what they need to do to recover. Likewise he has the ability to intervene on the person's behalf by communicating with the spirits. He may also prescribe herbs and aromatic incense, suggest an amulet, encourage prayers to figurines, or promote recitation of prayer cards. All can be purchased at folk religious stores called Botanicas.

If hospitalization is required, family is expected to be present and care for the individual. The patient takes a passive role. This may conflict with the nurse's belief that the patient should "do for himself." While the HCP is respected and held in high esteem, it is imperative to include family, extended family, priest, and santeros in planning care.

Health care in Prison

In the prison setting, safety and security dictate access to care. For HCPs, boundaries and the display of certain level of emotional protectiveness are integral to maintaining distance from inmates physically and emotionally. Medical care may be given a lower priority than safety, security or prison business. Care is given in a supervised setting with limited supplies. In order to assess an inmate's condition, it is vital that health staff recognize prevalent health issues for different ethnic groups. Puerto Ricans have the highest rate of asthma of any ethnic group. Gathering information from Carlito about his health history, beliefs about the cause of his asthma, as well as identifying prior effective treatments is integral to providing quality care. Showing an interest demonstrates respect and establishes the foundation on which trust can be built. In the article *Prison - Nurses Behind Locked Doors,* correctional nurses convey a frustration when caring for patients with chronic or high risk disease like Carlito because inmates "do not want to take care of themselves and/or not see a reason to do so."[81] While it is a challenge to work within the culture of prison, providing care and health education can have a positive outcome. When released from prison, inmates can take this knowledge with them.

Reflective exercise: Health Beliefs & Practices/Home Remedies/Healers
1. *Recognizing that there are limitations to interactions between HCP and patient within the prison setting – what are the most important aspects of Carlito's health beliefs and practices that need to be considered as relevant to care?*
2. *Are there triggers to his asthma episodes? Clinical? Emotional?*
3. *Are there ways to incorporate his home remedies and treatments into his care?*
4. *How do your beliefs about health, illness & treatment compare with his?*
5. *Where do you find common ground?*
6. *Does this change your approach?*

Religion

Spaniards brought more than language, literature and food preferences, to Puerto Rico, they also brought religion – Catholicism. Confession, penance, sacraments, holy days of obligation and rituals for birth, marriage and death were concepts foreign to the spiritual beliefs of the Taino Indians in 1493. Today, more than 85% of Puerto Ricans identity as Catholic. A relationship with God includes the belief that saints are emissaries that will plead their case. Roman Catholic priests are seen as sources of spiritual wisdom and support especially during times of illness, disability and death. Rituals such as praying and lighting candles serve as a protection against illness. Amulets and scapulars are worn to provide the assurance of good health – mentally, physically and spiritually. Additionally, rosary beads worn around the neck, prayer cards, holy water, aromatic lotions and prayers to the saints offer further protection. In the hospital setting, families may want these items placed at the bedside of their loved one to ward off any evil spirits. Prior to the removal of an amulet or other religious article worn by the patient, the family will contact the priest to provide a blessing.

Even those with a strong Catholic faith may also value and practice spiritism, which recognizes the good and evil found in the spirit world. Santeria and Espiritismo, are two forms of spiritism. They blend African, Native American and Catholic beliefs. Espiritismo proclaims that life is a spiritual test in which good conduct is rewarded through reincarnation of the spirit to a higher position in the celestial hierarchy. Santeria maintains that spirits (orishas) are assigned to each individual before birth to serve as guides and protectors in life.[82] It is believed that health issues, disharmony in relationships or spiritual problems need intercession by an indigenous healer. Santeros act as intermediaries with the spirit world. Powders, candles, incense and prayers may be used to enter the spirit world to communicate with the saints on their behalf.

Summary

Comparing and contrasting Puerto Rican and prison culture, we find common ground to establish rapport, build relationships and provide quality care. Loyalty and collaborative support found within all groups ensure health, protection and security. They are the building blocks that lead to respectful informative interactions and implementation of innovative health treatment options.

Culture Care Decisions and Actions

Acknowledge & Affirm
Loyalty & Respect
Family Interdependence

Discuss & Adjust
Family involvement
Identify initial symptoms
Visit by Priest and/or Santero

Collaborate & Change
Daily program - Peak flow
Scheduling routine appointments
Action with first symptoms

Resources

Arcay, D.A. (2011). The ethics of spiritual formation for a Christian Puerto Rican in a postmodern urban context. *Journal of Research on Christian Education.* 20:207-231.

Banghart, L. (2014). Is jail nursing safe? Working behind bars. Retrieved January 12, 2015 from www.Nursetogether.com

Berdahl, T.A., Stone, R. A. (2009). Examining Latino differences in mental healthcare use: The roles of acculturation and attitudes towards healthcare. *Community Mental Health Journal.* 45:393-403.

Brown, A., Patten, E. (2013). Hispanics of Puerto Rican origin in the United States, 2011. Pew Hispanic Center: Washington DC

Caballero, A.E. (2011). Understand the Hispanic/Latino patient. *The American Journal of Medicine.* 124:S10-S15.

Carlson, K. (2014). Correctional nursing: Interview with Marites Benito-Mateo RN, BSN, Caring for inmate patients in a guarded care environment. Retrieved January 12, 2015 from www.workingnurse.com

Campesino, M., Schwartz, G.E. (2006). Spirituality among Latinas/os implications of culture in conceptualization and measurement. *Advanced Nursing Science.* 29(1). pp. 69-81.

Carson, E.A. (2014). Prisoners in 2013. Bureau of Justice Statistics, National Prisoner Statistics Program. Washington DC: U.S. Department of Justice.

Dryden, P. (2003). Nursing behind locked doors. *Medscape Nurses.* 5(1). Hammer, C.S., Rodriguez, B.L., Lawrence, F.R., Miccio, A.W. (2007). Puerto Rican Mothers' beliefs and home literacy practices. *Language, Speech, Hearing Service School.* 38(3). pp. 216-224.

Hyman, R.C., Ortiz, J., Añez, L.M., Paris, M., Davidson, L. (2006). Culture and clinical practice: Recommendations for working with Puerto Ricans and other Latinas(os) in the United States. *Professional Psychology: Research and Practice.* 6:694-701.

Foster, J., Bell, L., Jayasinghe, N. (2013). Care control and collaborative working in a prison hospital. *Journal of Interprofessional Care.* 27:184-190.

Gannotti, M.E., Handwerker, W.P., Groce, N.E. (2001). Sociocultural influences on disability status in Puerto Rican children. *Physical Therapy.* 81:1512-1523.

Garcia-Preto, N. (2005). Puerto Rican Families. In McGoldrick, M., Giordano, J., Garcia-Preto, N. (Eds.) *Ethnicity and Family Therapy.* (2nd Ed.). New York: The Guilford Press.

Glaze, L.E. (2011). Correctional populations in the United States, 2010. *Bureau of Justice Statistics.* U.S. Department of Justice: Washington DC

Purnell, L.D. (2013). People of Puerto Rican Heritage. In Purnell, L.D. (Ed.) *Transcultural Health Care: A Culturally Competent Approach.* (4th Ed.). PA: F.A. Davis.

Lopez, I. (2008). "But you don't look Puerto Rican": The moderating effect of ethnic identity on the relation between skin color and self-esteem among Puerto Rican women. *Cultural Diversity and Ethnic Minority Psychology.* 14(2). pp. 102-108.

Martin, M., Beebe, J., Lopez, L., Faux, S. (2010). A qualitative exploration of asthma self-management beliefs and practices in Puerto Rican families. *Journal of Health Care for the Poor and Underserved.* 21:464-474.

Martinez, L.M., Padilla, M.B., Caldwell, C.H., Schulz, A.J. (2011). Examining the influence of family environment on youth violence: A comparison of Mexican, Puerto Rican, Cuban, Non-Latino Black and Non-Latino White adolescents. *Journal of Youth Adolescence.* 40:1039-1051.

Perry, J. (2010). Nursing in prisons: Developing the specialty of offender health care. *Nursing Standard.* 24(39). pp. 35-40.

Primm, A.B., Osher, F.C., Gomez, M.B. (2005). Race and ethnicity, mental health services and cultural competence in the criminal justice system: Are we ready to change. *Community Mental Health Journal.* 41(5). pp. 557-569.

Ramos, B.M. (2012). Psychosocial stress, social inequality, and mental health in Puerto Rican women in upstate New York. *Centro Journal.* 24(2). pp. 48-67.

Rivera, E.T., Wilbur, M.P., Roberts-Wilbur, J. (1998). The Puerto Rican prison experience: A multicultural understanding of values, beliefs, and attitudes. *Journal of Addictions & Offender Counseling.* 18(2). pp. 63-77.

Rivera-Soto, W.T., Rodriguez-Figueroa, L. (2012). Childhood obesity among Puerto Rican children: Discrepancies between child's and parent's perception of weight status. *International Journal of Environmental Research and Public Health.* 9:1427-1437.

Sherwood, C.H. (2014). Correctional facility nursing. Retrieved January 12, 2015 from www.minoritynurse.com

Stevenson, B. (2014). *Just Mercy: A Story of Redemption.* New York:Speigel & Grau.

Thompson, A.J. (1987). Standards for Health Services in Prison. Journal of the American Medical Association. 258(11). 1537. doi:10.1001/jama.1987.03400110119041.

Torres, S. (2013). Puerto Rican Americans. In Giger, J.N. (Ed.). *Transcultural Nursing: Assessment & Intervention.* (6th Ed.). Elsevier: California

Tucker, K.L., Mattei, J., Noel, S.E., Collado, B.M., Mendez, J., Nelson, J., Girffith, J., Ordovas, J.M., Falcon, L.M. (2010). The Boston Puerto Rican Health Study, a longitudinal cohort study on health disparities in Puerto Rican adults: Challenges and opportunities. *BMC Public Health.* 10:107-119.

Vangeepuram, N., Mervish, N., Galvez, M.P. Brenner, B., Wolff, M.S. (2012). Dietary and physical activity behaviors of New York City children from different ethnic minority subgroups. *Academic Pediatrics.* 12(6). pp. 481-488.

Wilper, A.P., Woolhandler, St., Boyd, J.W., Lasser, K.E., McCormick, D., Bor, D.H., Himmelstein, D.U. (2009). The health and health care of U.S. prisoners: Results of a nationwide study. *American Journal of Public Health.* 99(4). pp. 666-672.

Maeve's Story

Creating the Illusion ... | 19

Alcoholism - Irish Family

Maeve burps. Heading for her cashier job in the auto parts store, she jolts off the curb in a fog not unlike the one that engulfs the Golden Gate. She was lucky to land this job at McElvey's here in the City, and she is appreciative of Patrick for heading her in a positive direction so soon after her arrival. Margret and Thomas are proud of their mother too; they won't have to work behind a register though.

If only she felt clear-headed this morning.

Maeve has prayed to the Virgin about her drinking. She knows Mary must have been a teetotaler, even when she was dealing with a son who was a bit of an odd duck. Mary didn't rely on the bottle. Of course, Maeve doesn't either. She just feels more at ease after a belt or two.

"Sure hope I can find the right keys on the register."

Polly, the other woman in the office, is waiting when Maeve stumbles in. Polly has no children and little faith, but she was drawn immediately by Maeve's tall *tales and her combination of strength and vulnerability. Polly has a brother who is overly fond of Porter's too.*

"Morning, Maeve. McElvey left the overdue accounts for you to call. Third drawer on the left."
Getting no response, she continues,
"There's coffee in the pot, fresh-brewed. You OK?"
"Grand. Simply grand."

Maeve is still thinking of Margret and Thomas as she scans the accounts page dancing before her eyes. She knows her children will succeed in their new land. They are obedient offspring, schooled in the ways of the old country but eager to adapt; they are young enough. She wonders what sin it was that made the bottle paramount in her life---neglecting her lenten resolutions, resenting her blond and buxom cousin, giving in too quickly to Uncle Ed, having babies too soon? After all Patrick has done to gain her a foothold out here, she shouldn't be thinking this way. Luckily the veils of denial still obscure acknowledgement of any real problem

---

Reflective exercise: Alcoholism & Those in Denial
1. *Have you or someone in your family had problems with alcohol consumption?*
2. *If so, did it interfere with your relationship? In what ways?*
3. *Did that experience bias your opinion of patients who are alcoholic?*
    a. *Are you more sympathetic?*
    b. *Are you more critical or intolerant?*
3. *Does your image of what it means to be an alcoholic match with reality?*
4. *Do you routinely ask the CAGE questions of clinic or hospitalized patients?*

Alcoholism Rising

The *Summary Health Statistics for U.S. Adults: National Health Interview Survey, 2012,* cite the following statistics: over 52% of adults aged 18 years and older are regular drinkers; men consume more than women; with the highest percentage of drinkers being non-Hispanic White. From 2006 to 2012, 88,000 people have died from alcohol related illnesses. What constitutes a "drink"?

- 12-ounces of beer (5% alcohol content)
- 8-ounces of malt liquor (7% alcohol content)
- 5-ounces of wine (12% alcohol content)
- 1.5-ounces of 80-proof (40% alcohol content) distilled spirits or liquor[83]

Rates of alcohol consumption vary from state-to-state and country-to-country. Ethnic groups vary in their drinking as well, from a low percentage in Iran and Saudi Arabia to a high rate of intake in Luxembourg and Ireland. While the Irish are second in alcohol consumption internationally, they represent the highest prevalence of alcohol related problems. Irish women are less likely to drink than Irish men. However, among women from all ethnic groups, they have the highest alcohol consumption rate.[84]

There are varied hypotheses for increased alcohol consumption in the Irish. One may conjecture that it was the consequence of having an over dominant and manipulative Irish mother who ruled the family. As a result, drinking large quantities of alcohol offered a break from reality. The village pub provided the refuge and soon became the center of the community. Or possibly it was a result of the Great Potato Famine in the mid 1800s. It was a time of deep despair and, *the drink* helped alleviate the sense of instability and uncertainty. In the early 20th century many single Irish women emigrated to the United States, seeking employment. They broke the constraints of gender roles so ingrained in the Irish culture.[85] Drinking at the pub in America was acceptable for women. Still another theory is that increased alcohol consumption is related to a normative religious structure within the Catholic church. A study of Irish

American Catholics posits that alcohol consumption is reflective of a routinized cycle of rebellion (abusive drinking) and reinstatement (confession, forgiveness and re-incorporation into group life).[86] Unfortunately, stories portraying the Irish as heavy drinkers have lead to stereotyping and misconceptions.

Maeve had not thought her alcohol intake would affect her as it did her mother and grandfather. However, as a result of years of hardships and discrimination in Northern Ireland, and now as a new immigrant in the United States, her ability to cope with everyday life is waning. Still, she believes that her Catholic faith and the resilience of her Irish heritage will provide the strength to face this as well.

First a wee bit of history . . .

Life in Ireland was arduous. The never ending struggle dictated life choices. According to McGoldrick "for many centuries Ireland was dominated, oppressed, and exploited by the British. Irish history includes starvation, humiliation, and heartbreak on one hand, and a remarkable adaptive ability to transform pain through humor, fierce rebellious spirit, and courage to survive on the other."[87] Beginning in the 16th century, England ruled the island and created a deep division between Protestants and Catholics. Furthermore, they established laws which forbade Catholics from attending school, owning land, or applying for a position in military or civil service. Laws of discrimination prompted many to dream of a better life somewhere else.

Religious persecution and deplorable economic conditions in Ireland lead to the first wave of emigrants to the Virginia and Maryland colonies in the early 1600s. They did not receive a warm welcome and experienced discrimination both socially and politically. Yet, their values of religion, hard work, and education contributed to their new country. By the late 1770s, the Irish made up almost ten percent of the population in the United States. The second wave followed the Great Famine of 1845. The potato, a main staple for Irish families, was infected with a fungus and 50% of the crop was lost. It is said that between 1846 and 1850, the population of Ireland dropped by **two million**, one million to starvation and one million emigrated to North America.

From persecution and starvation in their home country, to discrimination and poverty in their new country, these immigrants proved loyal by enlisting to fight in the Civil War. In 1863, Congress passed The National Conscription Act which specified that unmarried men between the ages of twenty-one and forty-five were subject to a draft lottery. However, a loop hole in the law allowed wealthy men to "hire" a replacement for $300. Due to poor socioeconomic conditions, many Irish men answered those ads. They hoped that by this demonstration of allegiance and willingness to serve and die, that anti-Irish discrimination would end.

The turn of the century brought socioeconomic gains for the Irish. Unfortunately discrimination continued to plague them. My Irish grandfather told us stories of his emigration to California from County Cork at the turn of the century. He was a young lad of 6, but he remembers well being teased by the other children because of his accent. As an adult he frequently heard negative comments about the "flat-footed" Irish cop that patrolled his neighborhood. Nonetheless, his unwavering Catholic faith and church community sustained him and his family during those difficult years. Surprisingly, even at the age of 94, he continued to feel the pangs of inequities that cast a "dark cloud," as he would say, over his life.

According to the 2010 US Census Bureau, the number of U.S. residents who claimed Irish ancestry is 34.7 million, more than seven times the population of Ireland itself. The median income of Irish Americans is higher than median income for other households in the United States. Their poverty rate of 6.9% ranks among the lowest of all Americans.[88]

Cultural Beliefs and Values

Irish Americans are known to be family oriented, hard working, religious, and musical. These values, brought over during the waves of emigration, served to fortify their identity, their faith and their community. Upon arrival in the United States, they established Catholic churches throughout America. In addition to being the center for community activities, the church served as a resource in times of difficulty. While not much is known about Maeve, other than her current issue of alcoholism, one can consider that her Irish cultural beliefs and values are the cornerstone to her stability and safety. They provide her with the strength to face the difficulties in her life – job, co-workers, adult children and her addiction.

Cultural Beliefs and Values

Independence & Hard Work
Loyalty
Respect for the Elderly, the Priest & those in Authority
Religion
Family & Community
Folk & Religious Health Beliefs

Reflective exercise: Being Irish
1. *Which of these beliefs/values do you think is the most important to Mauve? Why?*
2. *Which one is most important to you? Why?*
3. *Which values would Mauve consider most helpful to deal with her alcoholism?*
4. *How would you incorporate these into your conversation? Into developing a plan of care?*

Communication

The Irish have a strong history of and value for the oral tradition. Storytelling, a famous Irish tradition, entertains those of all ages. "Think blarney, shenanigans and malarky" and you'll have a great story that engages all who listen. My grandfather told stories of his homeland replete with the "little people" and their "shenanigans."[89] We grew up being a "wee bit" leery of stormy nights when we "knew" the "little people" might come by and look inside our window. We made sure we were "tucked in our beds fast asleep" so as not to invite them in! Like many Irish, my grandparents had over time lost their accent, but when it came to storytelling the inflection on certain words added a "bit of the blarney" and drew our rapt attention. The power of some stories continue to influence my life today.

For the Irish, the use of humor and sarcasm is common. Humor, a great resource to cope with life's problems, is also used to manage uncomfortable situations. While appearing reserved in public, with family and friends the Irish are loud and demonstrative. Facial expressions add to the conversation. Embellishments add to the conversation. Moreover, verbal innuendos, ambiguity and metaphors convey a message as well. Eye contact is highly valued and an important aspect of conversation. It connotes a person is trustworthy, respectful, and honest. If eye contact is averted one may be viewed as guilty of some deed. Although displays of emotion or affection are limited in public, this same strategy is used when there is a dispute with a family member. The silence that follows a disagreement can lead to long term resentment. Relationships may be severed for a lifetime without a word.

During an appointment with the HCP, the Irish American patient may seem as verbose, exaggerating the presenting symptoms. However, it is important to note that this approach may serve to cover up or underscore something more serious. Woven in between the words is the true concern. Use of the phrase "I'll let you know" or "We'll see" or "Perhaps" may be used to express a "no" response. Our job is to find the message in the midst of the story. Take time to reflect back on what you've heard. Ask open and closed-ended questions and respect the response. It is in this venue that we glean the information needed to assess and plan care.

> *Reflective exercise: Communication & Storytelling*
> 1. *Are you a "get to the point person?"*
> 2. *If so, how do you manage lengthy dialogues that embellish and exaggerate?*
> 3. *Do you cut them off?*
> 4. *Do you listen patiently, but think "how much longer?"*
> 5. *If time were not an issue, would you be more open and inquisitive?*
> 6. *How would you validate Mauve's story & her perception of her condition?*
> 7. *Is it difficult for you to find common ground?*

Time Orientation

As we have seen throughout this chapter, the past plays a significant role in present thinking and conversation. Irish stories convey a strong sense of tradition. This translates to present day appreciation of family, community and good health. Their future orientation focuses on assuring prosperity and security for themselves and the next generation.

Family

Historically, one cannot view the Irish American family without acknowledging a history of oppression in their home country in which men were systematically deprived of a sense of place or power. It has been written that many *"turned to the drink"* to escape the day-to-day reality of poverty and oppression. As a result, women became dominate in marriage. The wife was expected to maintain the household with a focus and hope that her children would do better. Many single Irish women chose emigration, rather than marriage. There was an implicit reluctance on these newly immigrated women to marry.

However, couples today are more egalitarian. Together, they adhere to family values that include maintaining socioeconomic stability through hard work, promoting education for the children, and attaining professional accomplishments. Likewise, loyalty to family members is the core of stability in the home structure. As such, the elderly are provided for in their old age – financially and physically. They are sought out for their opinions and advice. Children are expected to demonstrate respect and obedience to their parents and elders. Rarely praised or made the center of attention, children are expected to be independent, self-reliant, and do well in school. Children may be thought of as good or bad, and parents may ignore the aspect of the child's behavior that does not fit in the designated role – "My Denny," "Poor Betty," "That Kathleen."[90] Siblings and cousins are close throughout a lifetime. The extended family is integral to the family structure as well. While they may not see each other frequently, they do get together for visits and are available for assistance when needed. Nonetheless, one does not want to rely on another too much as it may be considered a burden.

Health Practices

The Irish are a people of paradoxes. While enjoying a good time, they savor tragedy. They may boast and brag with confidence, yet believe that if something goes wrong it is a result of their sins. Although frequently joking, they seem to struggle always against loneliness, depression and silence, believing intensely that life will break your heart one day.[91] Problems are private matters, therefore Mauve may not seek care or counsel. It follows that if she can do the task at hand, she sees no need for an appointment with her HCP. Illness, whether attributed to guilt or sin or some self-fulfilling prophecy. is thought to be the result of some outside force. Ascribing an external locus of control is seen as a way of coping with physical or psychological problems. The belief is, that given enough time, the problem will resolve itself. The perception of illness may also be localized so to emphasize the cause. For example if the patient has symptoms involving the ears, eyes or mouth, it may be in response to a recent situation. The thought may be "what should I have heard?," "what should I have seen?," or "what should I have said?" These may have been some of Maeve's thoughts.

Since Maeve is able to go to work every day, she does not perceive her drinking to be a problem. Although her ability to function seems questionable, it's not enough of an issue, for her, to seek care. She would only go to the clinic as a result of an injury (motor vehicle accident, fall, or burn secondary to binge drinking) or perhaps to resolve issue with insomnia especially if interferes with her ability to work. Nevertheless, we know that a clinic appointment provides the opportunity to assess her current health, immunization status, screenings for pap smear and mammogram as well as her tobacco and alcohol consumption.

There are several effective screening tools used in the assessment of alcohol consumption. The most familiar is CAGE – an acronym that addresses intake. Her response to the questions may heighten her awareness of the problem. Does she feel the need to **C**ut down on drinking; "are others **A**nnoyed by your drinking;" does she feels **G**uilty about the drinking and does she need that first drink in the morning, the **E**ye opener, in order to start her day. Answering positive to more than two may meet the DSM-III (Diagnostic and Statistical Manual of Mental Disorders) criteria for abuse or dependence diagnosis.

Once the diagnosis is made, and she seems ready to stop drinking, you can work with her to develop a plan. An effective approach is one that focuses on the problem, is structured, brief, and goal-oriented. Alcoholic Anonymous (AA) is a support group that in many ways correlates with the Irish values of reliance. It has a spiritual component as well. It could serve as a social venue similar to that of the village pub as community. The concept of anonymity, an openness to strangers, correlates well with the practice of telling a stranger more intimate information than telling family members..

In addition Mauve could be experiencing depression or anxiety. If so, she most probably would not share that information on her initial visit. Perhaps, begin the conversation by asking her about her disruptive sleep cycle and how that impacts her ability to fulfill her work responsibilities. One effective assessment tool is The Hamilton Depression and Anxiety Rating Scale which includes the Short Sleep Index (SSI). This allows the HCP to assess both anxiety and insomnia. The SSI scale quantifies the main symptoms of sleep disturbance – difficulty falling asleep, staying asleep, early morning awakening, and poor sleep quality. Given that time for an appointment is limited, these screening tools are easy to use and brief to administer. And most importantly, it can give Maeve insight into her condition.

It is possible that Maeve has tried home remedies and participated in church rituals, hoping to end her alcohol addiction and depression. The Catholic Church provides rituals to deal with physical, emotional and mental health problems. These include blessings, wearing a scapula or medal, praying to the saints and lighting candles. Along with a belief in eating a balanced diet, exercising regularly and getting a good night's sleep, some other preventative measures consist of folk practices such as tying a bag of camphor around the neck to prevent flu; never looking in the mirror at night; closing closet doors to prevent evil spirits from entering the body; and never going to bed with wet hair. Folk treatments include drinking nettle soup to clear the blood, tying onion to the wrist or dirty sock around the neck to cure fever; drinking hot tea and lemon for a sore throat; eating raw onion or drinking hot tea with whiskey to cure a cold; and wrapping hot bread, sugar and soap in a linen cloth and placing it on an infection to cure boils.[92] These healing practices, passed down from one generation to the next, are still considered potent and beneficial today by many.

So how does one begin the conversation? Perhaps the HCP could open with a smile and handshake welcoming Maeve into the practice and then follow with open ended questions. What do you think caused you to be sick? What home remedies have you used? Have they been helpful? Finally, what is you greatest concern? This conversation establishes an interest and respect for her health beliefs and practices. Our ability to listen, to ask questions and to clarify misunderstandings helps establish rapport and hopefully assure the beginning of a trusting relationship. Together with the patient, we can develop a plan of care that incorporates some of her folk and religious practices.

> *Reflective exercise: Health Beliefs & Practices/Home Remedies*
> 1. *Acknowledging Mauve's family history*
>   a. *Did her grandfather or mother seek treatment – from whom? Healer, Priest, HCP.*
>   b. *Was it effective?*
> 2. *Which treatment, do you think, she'd like to try first?*
> 3. *If she's not open to a discussion of treatments – what's the next step?*
> 4. *Which aspect of her Catholic faith could be considered? Would you invite the priest to collaborate with you?*

Religion/Spirituality

Catholic, Protestant, Quaker, and Episcopalian are religious groups found in Ireland. Irish Americans are predominately Catholic. The church continues to play a dominant role in the Irish American culture. A source of strength in times of illness, disability, and death, these tenets remain a stable fortress on which to rely. Wearing religious medals helps maintain health, as well as provide comfort and protection. In our narrative Maeve "prays to the Virgin" about her drinking. Praying to the Virgin Mary and to saints who hold special powers (St Jude - patron of lost causes), infers an expectation that her petitions are heard and that prayers are answered. Reciting the rosary, which is usually done for a specific purpose, is another form of prayer. I remember when my Irish Mother declared that we, as a family, were going to say the rosary nightly. The reason – she was pregnant with triplets and wanted to ensure a safe delivery of three healthy babies. Every night after dinner for six weeks, we said the rosary. Not surprisingly, she delivered three healthy babies on her due date December 8th– the Immaculate Conception –a holy day in the Catholic tradition.

As HCPs it is important to acknowledge the reliance on religious beliefs by our patients. They influence one's decision on issues in health and illness. We could ask Mauve – "How do your religious beliefs (or your Catholic faith) help you during times of illness, stress, or disability?" If hospitalized, there are two additional questions we can ask – "Would she like to receive communion and would she like a visit from a priest?" This demonstrates our understanding and respect for her Catholic traditions and rituals. A visit by a priest assures that petitions are heard. The "Sacrament of the Sick," as it is known in the Catholic faith, is a ritual performed by the priest when one is seriously ill or facing impending death. This ritual includes anointing with blessed oil, communion (small unleavened wafer made of flour and water), and a blessing. It is thought that this rite promotes healing and comfort. Incorporation of religious practices acknowledges her faith, the power of prayer and healing.

Summary

Maeve has a strong belief in the power of the Virgin Mary. She has loyalty to her sons and does not want to show disregard for their concerns. Yet, she continues to cast a veil over the real issue of her inability to stop drinking. While her priest, her HCP and her family are supportive, revealing her weakness is not part of "how she was raised." However, with each visit we can offer her an opportunity to talk about life now and how it compares with life in Ireland. Helping her to find a wee bit of Ireland in the community is a good start. In addition, during the appointment, we can share with her results of CAGE and SSI – and ask for her thoughts. The insights that emerge may encourage her to face her issue of alcoholism and motivate her to seek treatment.

Culture Care Decisions and Actions

Acknowledge & Affirm
Family loyalty & Kinship
Resilience & Work Ethic
Religious Beliefs

Discuss & Adjust
Religious & Folk Rituals
Outside Support Groups
Dietary Intake

Collaborate & Change
Dependency on Alcohol
Exercise & Healthy Eating

Resources

Blackwell DL, Lucas JW, Clarke TC. (2014). Summary health statistics for U.S. adults: National Health Interview Survey, 2012. National Center for Health Statistics. Vital Health Stat 10(260).

Dedesma, R.K., Kallivayalil, D, Albanese, M.J., Eisen, J.C. (2014). A slow suicide: The seemingly infinite cycle of alcohol and trauma in a middle-aged woman. Harvard Review of Psychiatry. 22(1), 46-64.

Epstein EE, Fischer-Elber K, Al-Otaiba Z. (2007). Women, aging, and alcohol use disorders. *Journal of Women Aging* 19:31–48.

Leininger, M.M. (1991). *Culture Care Diversity and Universality: A Theory of Nursing.* National League for Nursing Press: New York.

Martin, C.M. (2013). Irish Americans. In Giger, J.N. (Ed.), *Transcultural Nursing: Assessment & Intervention.* Missouri: Elsevier Mosby

Mullen, K., Williams, R., Hunt, K. (1996) Irish descent, religion, and alcohol and tobacco use. *Addiction.* 91(2): 243-254.

McGoldrick, M. (2005). Irish Families. In M.M. McGoldrick, Gordiano, J., Garcia-Preto, N. (Eds.) *Ethnicity & Family Therapy.* (3rd. Ed.). New York: The Guilford Press.

O'Connor, G., (2012). Breaking the Code of Silence: The Irish and Drink. Retrieved 1.36.2015 from www.irishamerican.com

Perney, P, Rigole, H., Mason, B, Dematteis, M., Lehert, P. (2015) Measuring Sleep Disturbances in Patients with Alcohol Use Disorders. *Journal of Addictive Medicine.* 9(1): 25-30.

Perney P, Lehert P, Mason BJ. (2012). Sleep disturbance in alcoholism: proposal of a simple measurement, and results from a 24-week randomized controlled study of alcohol-dependent patients assessing acamprosate efficacy. *Alcohol: An International Biomedical Journal.* 47:133–139.

Rao, R., Wolff, K., Marshall, E.J. (2008). Alcohol use and misuse in older people: A local prevalence study comparing English and Irish inner-city residents living in the UK. *Journal of Substance Abuse.* 13(1): 17-26.

Rapple, B. (2010). Irish Americans. Retrieved October 2, 2014 from www.everyculture.com/multi/Ha-La/Irish-American

Rivest, J., Jutras-Aswad, D., Shapiro, P.A. (2013). Treating the "unhealthy alcohol user" on medical wards. *Journal of Psychiatric Practice.* Vol. 19 (3). 213-226.

Wilson, S. A. (2003). People of Irish Heritage. In Purnell, L.D., Paulanka, B.J. (Eds.). *Transcultural Health Care: A Culturally Competent Approach.* (2nd Ed.) PA: F.A. Davis.

Sammy's Story
Belonging . . .

20

Youth & Gangs

"Yeah, so what?"
The ER nurse, Ed Rosemund, is trying to ascertain exactly how Sam's upper lip got split so badly it needs stitches. Sam is wondering why he has to deal with this fruitcake instead of a nice curvy nurse. Ed tries again.
"You were wearing blue in 'the wrong part of town' and this big guy jumps you for no reason?"
"You got a problem with that?"
"Well, no, but it looks as if your lip does. Does your family know the cops sent you here to ER? Oh and by the way, it's 11AM on a Wednesday. School's still in session, right?"
No response from Sam. He's wondering why Jake and Trey, recent departees from the continuation school he hopes to attend when he's a teen, just laughed when they heard his story. Sam had strutted off through Red turf to hang out with his

homies. He'd gotten pretty close too before the fight came down---well, not a fight really; they call it an altercation or somethin' like that.

"And I could see Max on the corner going to tell the other Teals that I'd gotten thunked. I thought he was at least as good a friend as Oscar. Oscar the rat who told Ma I was skippin' school. Old ass-kissing Oscar even likes Rumsey Middle School, I can tell. F@#*in" freak!"

Ed tries again. He sees Sam's eyes tearing up.

"That lip must hurt. Bet it was a big guy you were fighting, if the angle of the blow is any indication. We do need to notify at least one parent, Sam. But no one else needs to know. Who would you like me to call before Dr. Rasmussen sees you?"

> *Reflective exercise: Perception versus Reality*
> 1. *Gang members – what image comes to mind?*
> 2. *Is there gang activity in your neighborhood or around your work place?*
> 3. *Can you look beyond the outward appearance when caring for a gang member?*
> 4. *What is your greatest concern?*

Gangs . . . From an Historical Perspective

We think of gangs as a new phenomena. In reality, they have been around for centuries. They served a purpose in the Middle Ages by performing socially acceptable functions such as "guardians of social morality," therefore assuring a decent and upright society. They worked in collaboration with, and had the support of, the local community. In the 1800s, in cities like New York and Chicago, socially marginalized youth formed gangs with the sole purpose of reaping economic benefits and being noticed. It offered a venue for the recently immigrated to make money and gain political standing. The Sugar House Gang, formed in the 1920s in Detroit, protected the Jewish merchants. Similarly, in other parts of the country, Italian, Irish, and Mexican youth formed gangs to ensure safety from outsiders. In the 1940s it was the Harlem gangs of New York City. In the 1960s it was the Black Panthers, Vice Lords, and the Black Liberation Army. They focused on social activism and addressed issues of racism, poverty and inequality. The attraction to become a member in a gang has a similar draw today – sense of purpose and belonging.

Today - Demographics & Definitions

Although gangs exist internationally, there is a greater level of study and research done on gangs in the United States. According to the National Youth Gang Survey 2004, there are more than 24,000 active gangs with 756,000 members in the United States. In the 2011 follow up survey, those numbers increased respectively to 29,900 and 782,000. Who are gang members? According to a recent national law enforcement survey done by the Department of Justice (DOJ), the ethnicity of gang members is 31% African-American, 47% Hispanic, 13% white, and 7% Asian. The results revealed that when individuals are more acculturated to main stream society, they are more likely to join a gang. Gangs provide a sense of personal empowerment in a society in which they feel they have none.[93]

A gang is defined as a collection of individuals bound by a commitment to an ideal. The DOJ and FBI provide a more extensive description of gang – a group of recurrently associating individuals or close friends with identifiable leadership and internal organization, identifying with or claiming control over territory in a community, and engaging either individually or collectively in violent or other forms of illegal behavior. In many situations, gang members have to prove their loyalty by committing such acts.[94]

Membership identification is divided into groups. The smallest group are called "Wannabe" members. Similar to our protagonist Sammy, they are early adolescents struggling with identity and place. They make up less than 10% of the membership. They "hang" with the gang to prove their allegiance. Regular gang members account for 40-50%. They readily self identify as members. Associate gang membership hovers at 20-30%, while hard core OG (Original

Gangsta) accounts for 10-20% of the group.[95] The following is a compilation of characteristics attributable to members.

Gang Members
- Interact frequently with one another
- May be involved in illegal activities
- Share common collective identity expressed in a gang name
- Express identity by adopting certain symbols
- Claim control over certain "turf"

Gang formation serves to maintain an economic base in the face of poverty. Moreover, according to Dr. Hugo Tapia, states the creation of a gang is "an attempt to regain power/control that was lost . . . to promote fear, intimidation toward the dominant culture . . to preserve economy of particular group when group is overpowered threatened by dominant culture."[96]

What's the draw?

For some, it is a belief in core values of honor, friendship, manliness, pride, recognition and self esteem. For others, it may be a response to a continual exposure to racism and discrimination, resulting in alienation from the main stream culture. Additionally, the desire to have a sense of family, safety, and identity – one that offers an ethnic or cultural similarity – is strong. Having control over their environment or "turf," is an opportunity to provide protection for family and neighborhood. Contributing to the well-being and safety of those they care about is the goal.

Core Values of Gang Members

Universally, there are common core beliefs and values in groups. Gangs are no exception. Membership requires adherence to these values. The research findings of Dr. Edith Morris (African American gangs) and Dr. Hugo Tapia (Hispanic gangs) highlight the importance of group values. Dr. Morris formed a relationship with African American gang members to learn the core values held in high esteem by their membership. The focus of her work was to discover and describe the culture care meanings and expressions of African American youth gang members. Her venture into the unknown was predicated on the belief that if we are to care for those involved in gangs, it is important for us in the healthcare field to understand, acknowledge, and incorporate these beliefs into our interaction with them. She identified the following values and beliefs:[97]

- Respect - giving and receiving as shown by:
  - Worthiness
  - Being Listened to
  - Concern for others
- Protection Surveillance & Trust (confidentiality)
  - Develop support systems to survive
  - Someone always watching out for them
  - Family & younger siblings
- Faith in (God)
  - Ameliorate harsh realities
  - Acknowledge that God is the reason one is still alive
  - Belief embedded in African American spirituality
- Love/Compassion

Dr. Hugo Tapia's study focused on creating a profile of the values of Mexican American (MA) gang members juxtaposed to Mexican adolescents who chose not to join gangs. He found that self-respect and social recognition were important to gang members while being loving, courageous, and capable held more value in the non-gang member. Dr Tapia's results highlight of values for MA gang members.[98]

- Honor - Respect - Pride
- Protect family honor & neighborhood
- Friendship
- Manliness
- Recognition & Self-esteem

> *Reflective exercise: Purpose & Focus*
> 1. *Are there similarities between your cultural values and beliefs and those found in the research by Drs. Morris & Tapia?*
> 2. *Which value would you select to create an open and welcoming dialogue with Sammy?*
> 3. *How could the standard approach of addressing the presenting problem lead to a discussion about home, school & peer groups?*
> 4. *Who else would you include in the conversation?*

Profile of a Perspective Member

What is the profile of a gang member? Generally they are more likely to be male than female, 90% to 10% respectively, and are between the ages of twelve and twenty-four. There is a direct correlation between gang membership and low socioeconomic status. Furthermore, the lack of parental involvement, exposure to violence, and limited social skills are factors that influence the decision to join a gang. Wannabes, like Sammy, are more likely to join when they feel a disconnect from family and friends at school, and are academically challenged. The following may contribute to a young person's desire to join a gang:[99]

- Increase incidents of physical fighting
- Feelings of hopelessness & lack of purpose in life
- Aggressive & rule breaking behavior
- In girls - Increased anxiety & depression
- Increased separation anxiety from mother
- Feelings of powerlessness & lack of control
    - Especially middle school students

> *Reflective exercise: Your patient's profile*
> 1. *Have you ever felt hopeless? Powerless? Separation anxiety?*
> 2. *Do any of your young patients match this profile?*
> 3. *What words would you expect to hear in this conversation?*
> 4. *Now that you have this information, how would you inquire about feelings of hopelessness, anxiety, lack of control at home, in school or around the neighborhood?*

Growth & Development in Adolescence

The period between the end of childhood and the beginning of adolescence can be a tumultuous time in a child's life. He is given more freedom and responsibility to make important decisions, yet feels as though he is being treated "like a child." It can be an ambiguous and contradictory time. This correlates well with the fifth stage of Erikson's Psychosocial Development – Ego Identity versus Role Confusion. It is during this time period that young people explore different roles which help them develop a personal identity. Acceptance by peer groups becomes essential. Youth, like Sammy, seek out groups that provide not only a sense of belonging, but also offer something greater than themselves. They look to older adolescents who, they assume, have the knowledge and the skill to navigate this maze of change. Gangs provide the acceptance and identity they are seeking.

There is a down side to this transition as well. According to Dr. Edith Morris, until the age of twelve, adolescents, who were gang members, expressed hope for their future. Unfortunately, her research found that by the age of thirteen, hope diminished and feelings of hopelessness and despair emerged. The focus became "stay alive and out of jail."[100]

Family

Living in an unsafe neighborhood and having unhealthily relationships with both parents and peers may affect how well they cope with challenging situations. Supportive families are probably the best protective factor for adolescents. While self disclosure to parents about neighborhood gang activity is a protective factor, peer pressure may take precedence. Some parents firmly believe and say to those who would listen – "my child would never join a gang." Unfortunately, many times they are the last to know because they ignore the signs. Good communication skills on the part of the parents, are essential in order to draw out the lure of gang involvement by their child.

HCPs must view the adolescent within the family context and recognize that family impacts the individual and the individual impacts the family. In addition, observing families as circular rather than linear, helps to maintain continuity in changing times. A focus on the individual strengths of each family member, coupled with encouragement to utilize resources that already exist within the family structure is an effective approach. Collaboration with parents, siblings and the youth ensures that all voices are heard, and that a variety of options are acknowledged. Identification of additional resources in the school, community and church can provide support.

Health Risk & Interventions . . . What We Need to Know

Sammy may have feelings of vulnerability and thoughts of – "don't trust docs" – during the appointment. Assuring him that everything said during the visit is confidential is the first step in the process. Discussion of physical health concerns provides a segue to having the conversation about emotional issues such as anxiety and depression which he may be reticent to discuss with parents and peers. In addition to addressing his healthcare concerns, we can show an inquisitiveness about his daily life – school, family, and any special interests he may have. We can ask: "How is he doing in school? What class do you like the most and why? Do you have any concerns about your home environment or the safety of your neighborhood?" These provide an opening to ask more in-depth questions such as, "Have you ever been exposed to violence?" We may be the only impartial person in his life to help him discuss those uncomfortable topics – drugs, sex, gangs, and relationship with his parents.

In the article, *"How physicians can help patients cope with trauma,"* Erin Allday shares results from a recent University of California at San Francisco research study that addressed exposure to violence and the effect on health. It suggests that these experiences can lead to mental health difficulties and substance abuse problems. The researchers posit that there is a direct correlation between exposure to violence and an individual's mental health, particularly anxiety, depression, and post-traumatic stress disorder (PTSD). Increased exposure to community violence can be a predictor that adolescent boys are more likely to join a gang and engage in violence after exposure to violence.[101] Acknowledging the correlation between depression and exposure to violence, we need to inquire about their exposure both in the past and the present. Continual exposure could lead to violence ideation especially when one feels inadequate, has low self-esteem or feels a sense of hopelessness. Dr Morris submits that *hope* is central to purpose and meaning of life and is inspired through the presence of a caring person. Can we be that caring person who extends a hand of hope?

> *Reflective exercise: Risk Assessment*
> 1. *Do you routinely assess for depression? Suicide ideation?*
> 2. *Do you ask about drug use? Alcohol use? Exposure to violence?*
> 3. *What tools do you use? Are they age/gender/culture appropriate?*
> 4. *What is your response when a patient says "no" I do not want to answer those questions?*
> 5. *How would you approach it differently?*

Interventions Plan of Care . . . The Keys to Success

Our responsibility is to listen and facilitate a discussion that centers on the health issues – physical and mental. The ambiance of the office setting and staff are integral to this process. It begins at the front desk with the receptionist who greets the youth by name, to the medical assistant who rooms him, and ultimately the HCP who builds on the former encounters to establish a safe, trusting environment. When we *Acknowledge and Affirm,* we create a non-judgmental and confidential environment. Appreciating his core values of respect, protection and surveillance of his neighborhood and younger siblings is crucial.

The Goal #1 for HCP:
- Create an accepting and safe caring environment
- Respect - listening non-judgmentally
- Assure confidentiality
- Provide recognition to promote well-being
- Reinforce their strength & skills (i.e. MA bilingual/bicultural)
- Recognize the value of protection for family & neighborhood
- Promote health screening for younger siblings.

Engaging in the *discussion* and demonstrating a genuine interest in his concerns –physical, mental, emotional and social – builds the bridge to understanding and rapport. Acknowledging of the barriers and biases he faces each day is a good segue to the conversation of gang involvement. Being open to his response displays a non-judgmental presence and may abate any anxious feelings of uncertainty and distrust. Affirming that his responses are familiar and normal may help the client to be more open to mental health screening and a provide a starting point in the relationship.

Goal # 2 for the HCP
- Promote collaboration
- Offer non-judgmental guidance
- Recognize socioeconomic status and impact on everyday life
- Acknowledge experience and impact of racism and discrimination
- Respect input of other gang members who may be present

Change is always the most difficult area to navigate regardless of age or health status. It challenges both HCP and patient to move away from the familiar and to trust that there are alternative healthcare options. Participation in screenings, such as a depression tool, demonstrates an openness on the part of the youth to gain awareness and a willingness to work toward change. Offering information about community venues, such as a Boy & Girls Club, Community Center or After School Program may provide inspiration to try something new. Safe havens, such as those listed, provide mentors who demonstrate new pathways and opportunities for growth.

Goal # 3 for the HCP
- Promote effective communication skills with parents
- Encourage parents/family to identify resources within their community - schools, community & churches
- Promote early mental health screening
- Work collaboratively with educators and gang members to identify ways to decrease violence

What else can we do . . . ?

We can work proactively to develop relationships with schools, neighborhood leaders, and community service organizations to address gang membership and activity. This collaboration provides a strong network of colleagues who offer a diversity of backgrounds, experiences and resources. It is through this process that we are visible to those who might seek our care and expertise. As we become more knowledgeable about current situations and are more open to discussions surrounding exposure to violence and gang activity, adolescents may be more inclined to listen and interact. Being active in the community and with those youth we encounter, we can offer a belief in change and give them hope for their future.

Resources

Allen, D. (2013). Walk on the wild side: Gang members need help too. *Mental Health Practice.* 16(9). pp. 6-7.

Branch, C. W. (1997). *Clinical Interventions with Gang Adolescents & Their Families.* Colorado: Westview Press.

Branch, C.W. (1999). *Adolescent Gangs: Old Issues, New Approaches.* Pennsylvania: Brunner/Mazel.

Clements, P.T. (2011). Youth gangs: Reason for concern. *Journal of Forensic Nursing.* 7:105-107.

Cregeen, S. (2008). Workers, groups and gangs: Consultation to residential adolescent teams. *Journal of Child Psychotherapy.* 34(2). pp. 172-189.

Dishion, T.J., Nelson, S.E., Yasui, M. (2005). Predicting early adolescent gang involvement from Middle School adaption. *Journal of Clinical Child and Adolescent Psychology.* 34(1). pp. 62-73.

Egley, A., Howell, J.C. (2013). Highlights of the 2011 National Youth Gang Survey. Washington, DC: U.S. Department of Justice. Office of Justice Programs.

Estrada-Martinez, L.M., Padilla, M.B., Caldwell, C.H., Schulz, A.J. (2010). Examining the influence of family environments on youth violence: A comparison of Mexican, Puerto Rican, Cuban, Non-Latino Black, and Non-Latino White adolescents. *Journal of Youth Adolescence.* 40:1039-1051.

Kelly, S.E., Anderson, D.G. (2012). Adolescents, gangs, and perceptions of safety, parental engagement and peer pressure. *Journal of Psychosocial Nursing & Mental Health Services.* 50(10). pp. 20-28.

Kelly, S.E., Anderson, D.G., Hall, L., Peden, A., Cerel, J. (2012). The effects of exposure to gang violence on adolescent boys' mental health. *Issues in Mental Health Nursing.* 33:80-88.

Kelly, S.E. (2010). The psychological consequences to adolescents of exposure to gang violence in community: An integrated review of the literature. *Journal of Child and Adolescent Psychiatric Nursing.* 23(2). pp. 61-73.

Martinez, L.M., Padilla, M.B., Caldwell, C.H., Schulz, A.J. (2011). Examining the influence of family environment on youth violence: A comparison of Mexican, Puerto Rican, Cuban, Non-Latino Black and Non-Latino White adolescents. *Journal of Youth Adolescence.* 40:1039-1051.

McNeil, S.N., Herschberger, J.K., Nedela, M.N. (2013). Low-income families with potential adolescent gang involvement: A structural community family therapy integration model. *The American Journal of Family Therapy.* 41:110-120.

Morris, E.J. (2012). Respect, protection, faith and love: Major care constructs identified within the subculture of urban African American adolescent gang members. *Journal of Transcultural Nursing.* 23(3). pp.262-269.

Morris, E.J., Fry-McComish, J. (2012). Hope and despair: Diverse voices of hope from urban African American adolescent gang members. *I International Journal for Human Caring.* 16(4). pp. 50-57.

Pacheco, H.R. (2011). *Gangs 101: Understanding the culture of youth violence.* Esperanza: Philadelphia.

Ryan, L.G., Miller-Loessi, K., Nieri, T. (2007). Relationships with adults as predictors of substance use, gang involvement, and threats to safety among disadvantaged urban high-school adolescents. *Journal of Community Psychology.* 35(8). pp. 1053-1071.

Scahn, M.H., Bossarte, R.M., West, B., Topalli, V. (2010). Alcohol and drug use among gang members: Experiences of adolescents who attend school. *Journal of School Health.* 80(7). pp. 353-360.

Tapia, H.A., Kinnier, R.T., MacKinnon, D.P. (2009). A comparison between Mexican American youth who are in gangs and those who are not. *Journal of Multicultural Counseling and Development.* 37:229-239.

Toy, C. (1992). A short history of Asian gangs in San Francisco. *Justice Quarterly.* 9(4). pp. 647-665.

U.S. Government. (2015). Brief Review of Federal and State definitions. Retrieved December 20, 2015 from www.nationalgangcenter.gov.

National Institute of Justice (2011). What is a gang? Definitions. Washington, D.C.: U.S. Department of Justice. Office of Justice Programs.

Diversity & Inclusion... The Best of All Worlds | 21

Our Nation derives strength from the diversity of its population and from its commitment to equal opportunity for all. We are at our best when we draw on the talents of all parts of society, and our greatest accomplishments are achieved when diverse perspectives are brought to bear to overcome our greatest challenges.

President Barak Obama
Executive Order 13583
August 18, 2011

Over the past decades, the term diversity has become background music to most people. A recent NPR program highlighted a study on the efficacy of diversity programs over the past 25 years, and callers' comments seemed split between the need for, and the effectiveness of, such programs. Over half indicated an irrelevance for them personally. Many thought "it was a waste of their time and did not apply to them," or "they'd already attended one in the past so no need to revisit as they knew everything." However, the guest researcher made a strong point – the most successful programs were ones that made the information applicable to their workplace. For those working in healthcare, understanding how another's (colleague or patient) cultural values and beliefs influence decisions and actions results in more respectful interaction, collaboration, and improved health outcomes.

As President Obama stated, we are a nation of immigrants and that continues today. Tech companies and universities recruit the "best and the brightest" by assisting new hires to secure the coveted H1 Visas. Hospitals extend invitations to Registered Nurses in the Philippines and parts of Africa. CEOs and Personnel Directors travel to those countries to offer perks such as housing, travel and licensure. As a result, hospitals and clinics are a collective of people of varying ages, ethnicities, gender, skill level and education. Though diverse, there is one missing link – inclusion. Are we interested in another's perspective? Their experience? Or are we just filling vacancies?

Working collaboratively to provide quality care invites opinions and ideas from the diversity of staff members. It helps to assure that we will meet the needs of patients and families. As with an orchestra, it takes a variety of instruments to create a musical masterpiece. While a symphony hall appears significantly different than the health care setting, it does provide a metaphor for embracing diversity and promoting collaboration. Both lead to team work, quality patient care, and good health outcomes for patients. In addition, an inclusive environment results in lower turnover rates, respectful relationships and increased staff and patient satisfaction. Most importantly, it encourages input from all the voices at the table. As a result, creativity thrives.

Culture of Inclusion

When we talk about culture, we usually associate it with an ethnic group's values, beliefs, and ways of living in the world. Thus it follows that in order to create an environment of inclusion, the values and beliefs of all groups must be known and respected. In addition, healthcare organizations have a "culture" as well. Ideally their values are reflected in their vision and mission statement. Think about your place of employment – does it promote a culture of inclusion, one in which an employee's input and perspective is encouraged and valued?

Consider the following key elements of an inclusive environment: equality, trust built on cooperation and reciprocal recognition, respect, and openness to different perspectives.[102] It has been shown that "diverse groups that include a multitude of perspectives and backgrounds fare better at solving problems than a homogeneous group.[103] Acknowledging diversity among employees and recognizing how individuals process information and make decisions, is vital to successful group collaboration.

An Inclusive Culture Values and Promotes

- Diversity
- Equality, trust and respect
- Creative Innovation
- Employee participation
- A welcoming environment

So What Gets in the Way?

The central barriers to creating an inclusive environment: prejudice, bias and discrimination. Hidden beneath are issues of power, authority, and control displayed as unequal distribution of job assignments, advancement, and scheduling. Seems harsh? Yet this is reality – an unspoken reality. Furthermore, discrimination in age, gender, ethnicity and seniority are on the list as well. The end result is distrust, and for some, a "why bother" attitude. Why bother to raise the issue? Why bother to apply for the managerial position? Why bother to voice concerns about bullying and pressure to accept heavy assignments? Hence, perception is regarded as reality.

What is prejudice? It is a bias, not based on fact. For many, these biased beliefs tacitly provide a sense of entitlement to elevate one's status and ego. While we may not want to admit our prejudices, we all have them. We rarely, if ever, would verbalize such thoughts in a mixed group. Unintentional or not, our prejudices and biases lead to discriminatory acts in our work environment.

Carol Tutus (2014) highlights four forms of workplace discrimination: isolate, small group, direct institution and indirect institutional. Each perpetuate practices that devalue another individual. Generally, workplace discrimination involves employees being evaluated according to their age, ethnicity or gender, rather than their skill level or the actual performance criteria. *Isolate discrimination* occurs as suggested, an isolated incident. In this situation it may be a patient refusing care from a particular nurse. One study found that more than 50% of Asian nurses and 66% of Black nurses experienced this form of discrimination. *Small group discrimination* occurs when the dominant group in the unit works to intentionally disrupt a staff member's day, by making a nurse feel invisible, discounting his skills, ultimately causing him to question his abilities to provide quality patient care. Unfortunately, if left unchecked this can lead to bullying, thus having an emotionally negative effect on the person as well. The end result – increased stress, self-doubt and job dissatisfaction. *Direct discrimination* focuses on wages, advancement, workload, requirement of overtime, weekend scheduling or denial of request for a day off. *Indirect institutional discrimination* is embedded in the culture of the organization and leads to an intangible sense of prejudice. Though not directly visible, it is ingrained in the unspoken. By allowing each of these discriminatory practices to continue the recipient of such discrimination cannot work to their highest potential, thus the organization loses out on the contributions of this person. [104]

Focus groups, educational seminars, review of policies, and a critical look at the distribution of power and how it is used to perpetuate discriminatory practices are ways to start the discussion. In the process of creating a culture of inclusion in which everyone is valued for their expertise and insights, issues of bias, prejudice and discrimination must be addressed. Valuing the contributions of all ensures fairness and justice. Workforce diversity is not accomplished by meeting the quotas of personnel hired, but rather by the opportunities each staff member has to participate fully in the workings of the institution.

Finding your voice . . . Hearing Another's

Understanding the concept of inclusion, and putting it into practice, requires a willingness to embrace the unknown and to learn the social skills needed to create this reality. Two significant elements that facilitate effective communication in an inclusive environment are Neurolinguistic Programming and Social Neuroscience. ***Neurolinguistic Programming*** focuses on how we take in and encode information. It is thought, when used effectively, rapport and trust can be fully realized. The premise is when we mirror another's style of communication, style and we seek clarification and ask questions, we gather more pertinent information in which to make accurate health assessment. *Neuro* reflects how we take in and encode information – seeing, hearing, feeling, taste and smell. For example a person who takes in information visually usually answers questions by describing a picture and uses phrases such as "I *see* what you mean." An auditory person describes sounds and says something like "*Sounds* okay to me." A feeling person describes emotions. The *linguistic* element refers to a person's style of communication – speed, tone, volume and pitch. *Programming* correlates to the way a person organizes their ideas and actions to produce desired results. The next time you are in a conversation try mirroring your patients or colleagues stance and style. The result–rapport is established and trust is built.

Neurologic	Visual	Auditory	Feeling
Eye Cueing	Looks up & to an angle	Looks to the side	Looks down & to an angle
Words	Describe picture	Describe sounds	Describes emotions
Response	"I see what you mean" "How does it look to you" "We see eye to eye" "That looks good to me"	"Sounds okay to me" "How does that sound to you" "That rings a bell"	"I feel like" "How does it feel to you" "I'll get in touch with you"

Figure 20-1 Neurolinguistic Programming

Social neuroscience addresses how people relate to each other. Brain association, thoughts, threats and rewards provide insight into why people respond to a given situation in a particular manner. The focus is on social behavior, specifically how one minimizing threats and maximizing rewards. David Rock developed the SCARF model, an acronym for Status, Certainty, Autonomy, Relatedness and Fairness – all considered social domains. The goal is to bring awareness to an otherwise non-conscious process, thus helping to minimize threats and maximize rewards. It is an opportunity for an individual to understand the previous responses to a given situation, to re-evaluate that response, and to change the current reaction to one that is more positive.[105]

- Status - one's relative importance to others
- Certainty - forecasting the future
- Autonomy - provides an ability to control and make decisions
- Relatedness - ability to interact with others in a safe venue
- Fairness - impression of a fair exchange between people

Each domain correlates to a portion of the brain that influences our social interactions. When activated, a response is triggered – avoidance (threat) or approach (reward). Understanding this concept gives us an "aha" moment in which to understand our reaction. Now instead of reacting, we can either change our response or design our interaction to minimize the threat or maximize the reward. For example if you have a tendency to micromanage your staff, their autonomy is threatened. What could you do to change that into a reward? For starters you could avoid intervention, encourage independent thinking, and support their decision-making. The result – you've tapped into their internal reward. It is synonymous with receiving an excellent performance appraisal.

Challenges

Oh yes, there are many challenges that come with creating this ambience. Three identifiable factors are the lack of perceived need by administration, perceived lack of finances, and apathy of employees. So where to start? It begins with leadership's willingness to evaluate the current system, and embrace and value the concept of inclusion. While giving the proverbial nod to inclusion, administration may be unconvinced of the cost benefit to the organization. Furthermore, they may be hesitant to "give up their power" to control and monitor outcomes.

From an employee perspective they've "heard it all before" and perhaps view this as just another "feel good" presentation that they are required attend. Based on prior experiences, this program may not be viewed as credible, but rather "a waste of their time" – they have patients who need their attention and care. Redesigning the approach, from a mandatory attendance at a large group seminar to small discussion groups soliciting employee input, may be a more effective venue. Change, in any manner, requires a willingness on everyone's part to reassess the status quo and rethink the basic assumptions previously held. The challenge, therefore, is to convey the benefits to all who participate and to get them to "buy in." Change requires a willingness to alter our previous beliefs and thoughts.

The move toward a collectivistic or group approach signals an openness by leadership to listen to those voices rarely heard in the process. An administrative shift from "making decisions about change" to gathering "group input" is a paradigm shift in thinking and doing. Just as important is allocation of time and resources dollars. Does the current budget reflect resources necessary for both management and staff to learn about the benefits and challenges of creating an inclusive environment? If not, then perhaps developing a strategic plan that includes goals, objectives, time and resources is the first step. Planning is a cornerstone to success.

Promote the Value of Inclusion

Think about an organization or institution that values diversity and inclusion. What does that look like? Is it free from judgement, harassment, and disrespect? Does it promote collaboration, open communication and equal rights for everyone? Inclusive work environments acknowledge differences, affirm each person's contribution, and encourages staff to voice opinions and offer suggestions. A trusting and respectful environment facilitates meaningful discussions.

So how can your institution promote collaboration and encourage employees to contribute their expertise. The first step is **recognition**! Acknowledge that everyone's perspective and experience is valid and crucial to the discussion. This message communicates value and purpose – internally to staff and externally to the community. Diversity within the group can provide solutions that may not have been previously considered. It is through this process that previously marginalized voices are heard and supported. What a concept!

Key elements to create an inclusive environment:

- Mission statement and vision articulates the value of diversity and inclusion

- A rationale for diversity and inclusion - how do we benefit from a diverse and inclusive workforce?

- Ensure representation from all groups (age, ethnicity, gender, skill and education) and departments
- Objectives are stated clearly – how we plan to meet that goal of a diverse and inclusive workforce

- Accountability - who is responsible and how do we measure it?

- Recognition for being part of the process

- Assessment - measurable criteria - did we make it?

- Resources - identification of monies and resources (staff and other) to achieve the goal and implement the plan

A realistic plan takes into account that the given plan may not follow a straight line. Acknowledgement of minor setbacks and change in direction should be built into the process. And most importantly, all information must be disseminated to staff in a timely manner. The assessment models and tools listed in the next section serve as a foundation from which to build.

Summary

It is through this process of promoting diversity and inclusion that the organization's vision and mission statement come alive. What was once considered a good adage, now takes on meaning and substance. Diversity coupled with inclusion recognizes and values each person's contribution to the process. Voices reflective of various ethnic, gender, religious and age groups assure that change takes a broader view of the setting and provides a potpourri of possible solutions. Workforce diversity celebrates individual attributes and inclusion helps the organization meet the needs of staff, patients and their families and community.

Assessment & Tools

There are a variety of matrixes to choose from when assessing diversity and inclusion within an institution. Each of the following offer a method/plan to increase diversity and create an inclusive environment. Some focus on the individual and others on organization. The individual assessment is integral to understanding how diversity correlates with everyday patient care, family interactions, and colleague encounters. The organizational assessment is viewed from a systemwide approach which includes such aspects as personnel policies, performance appraisals, orientation programs and educational venues.

Listed below are some assessment tools to consider. Each should to be viewed within the context of the organization's goal and objectives and budget constraints to determine which one best fits the needs.

Diversity & Cultural Proficiency Assessment Tool for Leaders - composed of an easy to use assessment checklist which identifies the diversity of community, patient care, workforce, and leadership, followed by clearly stated action steps and cases studies. An extensive bibliography is included. This assessment tool was developed as a collaborative effort by the American Hospital Association, the National Center for Healthcare Leadership, the American College of Healthcare Executives and the Institute for Diversity in Health Management. www.aha.org

Balanced Scorecard in Health Care is based on the Kaplan & Norton Balanced Scorecard, and modified for healthcare. It has a development and community focus on human resources, patient satisfaction, clinical utilization and outcomes. In addition it includes quality of care outcomes and assessments. It encourages stakeholders to identify metrics to measure performance, thus linking the organizations vision, values and core principles to day to day operations. As a result all members of the team make a difference at the point of clinical services across a continuum. (Henry Ford Healthcare System - Sahney; JCAHO employee benefit plan review; DHHS mental health services)

Intercultural Development Inventory (IDI) is a theory based tool used to assess an individual's and/or organization's intercultural competence. It is an opportunity for staff to recognize their cultural perspective toward others, identifying similarities and differences, and then learn to modify that approach in everyday interactions. These insights help determine next steps to understanding the impact of current systems and encounters and opportunities for change. www.idiinventory.com

Resources

American Hospital Association. (2004). Strategies for leadership. Does your hospital reflect the community it serves? A Diversity and Cultural Proficiency Assessment tool for leaders. *Journal of Health Administration Education.* July/ August. pp. 1-23.

American College of Healthcare Executives. (2013). The healthcare executive's role in fostering inclusion of LGBT patient and employees. *Healthcare Executive.* May/June. pp. 113-115.

Bensimon, E.A. (2004). The diversity scorecard: A learning approach to institutional change. *Change.* January/February. pp. 45-52.

Burnell, Y. (2015). Corporate Diversity Programs Must Be Inclusive to be Successful. *Public Relations Tactics.* February. pp. 9.

Department of Defense. (2012). Diversity and Inclusion Strategic Plan. pp. 1-15. Retrieved January 3, 2015 from www.whitehouse.gove/the-press-office/2011/08/18/executive-order-establishing-coordinated-government-wide-initiative-prom.

Escallier, L.A., Fullerton, J.T. (2009). Process and outcomes evaluation of retention strategies within a nursing workforce diversity project. *Journal of Nursing Education.* 48(9). pp. 487-494.

Evans, A. (2007). Are the walls really down?: Best Practices in Diversity Planning and Assessment. ASHE Higher Education Report. 33(1). pp 89-102

Goodman, N.R. (2013). Taking diversity and inclusion initiatives global. *Industrial and Commercial Training.* 45(3). pp 180-183.

Homan, A.C., Hollenbeck, J.R., Humphrey, S.E., Knippenberg, D., Ilgen, D.R., Van Kleeg, F.A. (2008). Facing differences with an open mind: Openness to experience, salience of intragroup differences, and performance of diverse work groups. *Academy of Management Journal.* 51(6). 1204-1222.

Kirch, D.G., Nivet, M. (2013). Increasing diversity and inclusion in medical school to improve the health of all. *Journal of Healthcare Management.* 58(5). pp. 311-313.

Lincoln, B. (2009). Reflections from Common Ground: Cultural Awareness in Healthcare. Eau Claire, WI: PesiHealthcare

Moceri, J.T. (2014). Hispanic nurses' experiences of bias in the workplace. *Journal of Transcultural Nursing.* 25(1). pp. 15-22.

Obama, B (2011). Executive order-establishing a coordinated government-wide initiative to promote diversity and inclusion in the federal workforce. *Federal Register.* 76(163). pp. 52847-49.

Pearson, A., Srivastava, R., Craig, D., Tucker, D., Grinspun, D., Bajnok, I., Griffin, P., Long, L., Porritt, K., Han, T., Gi, A.A. (2007). Systematic review on embracing cultural diversity for developing and sustaining a healthy work environment in healthcare. *International Journal of Evidence-Based Healthcare.* S: 54-91.

Peters, P., Bleijenbergh, I., Poutsma, F. (2010). Towards a new culture of work-place inclusiveness: the Dutch case. *Equality, Diversity and Inclusion: An International Journal.* 29(5). pp. 532-533.

Pless, N.M., Maak, T. (2004). Building an inclusive diversity culture: Principles, process and practice. *Journal of Business Ethics.* 54: 129-147.

Reese, C. H., Rowell, P. (2009). Diversity and inclusion. *Financial Executive.* January/February. pp. 52-55.

Rock, D. (2008). SCARF: a brain-based model for collaborating with and influencing others. *NeuroLeadership Journal.* 1: 1-9.

Steward, M., Crary, M, Humberd, B. (2008). Teaching value in diversity: On the folly of espousing inclusion, while practicing exclusion. *Academy of Management Learning & Education.* 7(3). pp. 374-386.

Sweeney, P. (2009). Attributes of diversity and inclusion. *Financial Executive International* November. pp. 18-21.

Thomas, B. (2014). Health and health care disparities: The effect of social and environmental factors on individual and population health. *International Journal of Environmental Research and Public Health.* 11:7492-7507.

Tuttas, C. (2014). Perceived racial and ethnic prejudice and discrimination experiences of minority migrant nurses: A literature review. *Journal of Transcultural Nursing.* pp. 1-7.

van Dick, R., van Knippenberg, D., Hagele, S., Guillaume, Y.R., Brodbeck, F.C. (2008). Group diversity and group identification: The moderating role of diversity beliefs. *Human Relations.* 61(10). pp. 1463-1492.

Villarruel, A., Washington, D., Lecher, W.T., Carver, N.A. (2015). A more diverse nursing workforce. *American Journal of Nursing.* 11(5). pp. 57-62.

Wilson, D. (2007). From their own voices: The lived experience of African American registered nurses. *Journal of Transcultural Nursing.* 18(2). pp. 142-149.

Wolf, A.C., Ratner, P., Robinson, S.L., Oliffe, J.L., Hall, L.M. (2010). Beyond generational differences: A literature review of the impact of relational on nurses' attitudes and work. *Journal of Nursing Management.* 18: 948-969.

U.S. Office of Personal Management. (2011). Government-wide diversity and inclusion strategic plan 2011. Office of Diversity and Inclusion. pp. 1-8

Closing thoughts... | 22

Whether striving for cultural competence or creating a more inclusive environment, the goals are the same – quality patient care that eliminates health disparities. Cultural knowledge and skills enhance our interactions with patients, families, colleagues and community. It is through this process of competence and inclusion that we gain a deeper and broader understanding of another's perspective. In the past, differences lead to misunderstanding and conflict. Now we recognize that these differences are opportunities to find common ground. As a result, we have a new appreciation and respect for another's way of living in the world.

Where to from here? Think of some of the ways that you could inspire colleagues to embrace and value diversity, cultural competence, and inclusion. Now, consider your organization's current policies and procedures – do they reflect those values? What is missing? Are there standards of care for the diverse populations you serve? Is providing culturally competent care a point of discussion during seminars and orientations?

Now that You Know

Rather than a mandated directive from administration to fill those gaps, it may be advantageous to begin the dialogue at the department level, perhaps at a staff meeting. This setting provides a comfortable venue for staff to discuss cultural competence and inclusion and how it influences patient care. Encourage staff to share stories in which their cultural beliefs, values and practices may have conflicted with their patient and family's view. Differences in expectations of patient involvement in care and family perception may add to tension and misunderstanding. Sharing narratives increases an awareness that we all have experienced feelings of frustration and many times lacked the cultural knowledge and skills to address the issue.

Consider the dilemma faced by the Physical Therapy department at a local hospital. Their problem was two fold – their Mexican American patients were not returning for follow up appointments, and when they did, they were accompanied by several family members. The physical therapist shared that they did not allow family members into the physical therapy room. It was policy! The result – patients stopped returning for their follow up visits. An inservice on the Mexican American cultural values, beliefs and practices as related to health care was held. Recognizing the value of family and the importance of their presence at the appointment, the physical therapist began to invite family to remain in the room with their loved one. The outcome – increase in compliance and speedier recovery.

Designing a program - Making it Inspirational & Relevant

The ubiquitous words – diversity, inclusion, competence and culture – have been become "white noise" to many in the healthcare field. As a result, attempts to promote diversity training have received an apathetic response. However, when a presentation is innovative, inspirational, participatory and applicable, attendees are more likely to value the information. Think for a moment. If you could design a program that would entice staff to attend, what would it look like? Perhaps one with more interaction, real-life scenarios, and clear application to practice might come to mind. A template for a Cultural Awareness & Competence seminar found in the appendix can be easily adapted to any venue – half day, full day or one hour. It's all about creativity – meeting the needs of staff without taking time away from patient care.

The cornerstone to a successful program lies with the planning committee and the freedom to "think outside the box." Equally important is committee membership. Does the group represent the organizations workforce in age, ethnicity, gender, and occupation? Each affirmative answer increases the likelihood of a successful program. The more diverse, the more reflective of your staff and patient population, the more credible the program. So, gather an eclectic group to create an inspiring and innovative program that speaks to overflow crowds!

If you are reading this now, then you are already thinking to yourself – who are the key people to approach and what resources are available to make this educational program a reality? Key to the success of such a venture is 'buy in' from Administration. If they espouse a similar vision and believe in the values diversity, cultural competence and inclusion, then monies will likely be allocated for educational training, consultants and staff time. Furthermore, having resources such as *Further Reflections from Common Ground: Cultural Awareness in Healthcare,* available on each unit may serve as an impetus for conversations about culture and care that otherwise would not have taken place. Be the voice of the most vulnerable and the champion of their needs. Your journey continues . . .

Appendix

Diversity & Inclusion Assessment Tools - Organizational & Individual

*Each should to be viewed within the context of the organization's goals and objectives, timeline and budget.

Cultural Competence Health Practitioner Assessment developed by the National Center for Cultural Competence through Georgetown University. The focus includes six sections: Values and Beliefs Systems, Cultural Aspects of Epidemiology, Clinical Decision Making, Life Cycle Events, Cross Cultural Communication and Empowerment/Health Management. These areas are used in conjunction with practitioner self-assessments looking specifically at cultural and linguistic competence.
www.gucchd.georgetown.edu/nccc/selfassessment.html

Cultural and Linguistic Competence Policy Assessment (CLCPA) developed by the National Center for Cultural Competence focuses on supporting and promoting cultural and linguistic competence in community health centers. In addition it reviews utilization and access to care with the goal of ending health disparities.
www.clcpa.infor/

Diversity & Cultural Proficiency Assessment Tool for Leaders - composed of an easy to use assessment checklist which identifies the diversity of community, patient care, workforce, and leadership, then follows with clearly stated action steps, and cases studies. An extensive bibliography is included. This assessment tool was developed as a collaborative effort by the American Hospital Association, the National Center for Healthcare Leadership, the American College of Healthcare Executives and the Institute for Diversity in Health Management.
www.aha.org

Balanced Scorecard in Health Care: based on the Kaplan & Norton Balanced Scorecard, and modified for health care. The development and community focus, human resources, patient satisfaction, clinical utilization and outcomes, and modified to include quality of care outcomes and assessment. Encouraging stakeholders to identify metrics to measure performance, thus linking the organizations vision, values and core principles to day-to-day operations. As a result, all members of the team make a difference at the point of clinical services across a continuum.

www.jsofian.files.wordpress.com/2006/12/use-of-bsc

Intercultural Development Inventory (IDI) – a theory-based tool used to assess an individual and/or organization's intercultural competence. It is an opportunity for staff to recognize their cultural perspective toward others, identifying similarities and differences, and then to modify that approach into their everyday interactions. The insights help determine next steps to understanding the impact of current systems and encounters and opportunities for change.

www.idiinventory.com

Improving communication – improving care is one of several tools offered through the American Medical Association (AMA) Ethical Force program toolkit. The focus of this tool is to assist the health care institutions to meet the needs of a diverse population. With a clear focus on promoting effective communication with staff, patients and communities, it takes into account culture, language, and literacy levels. The toolkit includes assessment surveys and protocols to guide the organization to achieve results.

www.EthicalForce.org

Conducting a Cultural Competence Self-Assessment is a tool designed by Dennis Andrulis from SUNY/Downstate Medical Center in Brooklyn, NY in collaboration with others in the field. This self-assessment tool to help organizations audit cultural competence in providing health care. It offers understanding of the ethical and cultural makeup of its patients, families and staff. This tool helps to assess the current communication between staff and patient/family is effective. It aids the organization to send a message to the community that it values and celebrates diversity.

www.erc.msh.org/provider/andrulis.pdf

The Cultural Competence Self-Assessment Protocol for Health Care Organizations and Systems is another tool developed by Dennis Andrulis and colleagues. This particular tool builds on the Georgetown University Child Developments Center's Continuum of Cultural Competency. The protocol expands the Georgetown University Child Development Center's Continuum of Cultural Competency. It can be used by the HCP, health organizations and departments to assess cultural competence. The four areas of cultural competence focuses on an institutions relationship with community; administration's relationship with staff; inter-staff relationship and patient/provider exchanges.
www.erc.msh.org/mainpage.cfm?file=9.1g.htm&module=provider&language=Eng

Race Matters: Organization Self-Assessment is provided by the Annie E. Casey Foundation. The questionnaire focuses on staff competencies and organizational systems as it relates to racial equity. It provides suggestions to follow up steps and other instruments/assessments to build awareness.
www.jdaihelpdesk.org/Docs/Documents/JDAI%20Inter-Site%20Conference%202006/organization_self_assessment.pdf

Self-Assessment for Cultural Competence developed by the American Speech Language Hearing Association features a web-based tool to assist in evaluating current cultural competence with a focus on improving service. It includes checklists, assessment tools and questionnaires. In addition, it aids in the review of policies, procedures and assessment of changes that may need to occur as it relates to the demographics of a culturally and linguistically diverse community
www.asha.org/about/leadership-projects/multicultural/self.htm#ccc

One Size Does Not Fit All: Meeting the Needs of a Diverse Health Care Population develop by Wilson-Strokes and colleagues is a detailed report that provides a framework and assessment tools for healthcare facilities to promote providing care for their diverse patient population. It encourages institutions to assess the needs of the community served and determine how they are being met currently. Suggestions such as assessments, monitoring, identification of barriers, review of mission statements and what is currently being offered educationally to staff.
www.jointcommission.org/assets/1/6/HLCOneSizeFinal.pdf

Indicators of Cultural Competence in Health Care Delivery Organizations: An Organizational Cultural Competence Assessment Profile developed by the Lewin Group Inc., Health Resources and Services Administration, Office of Minority Health and Office of Planning and Programming. It focuses on developing an analytical framework for assessing cultural competence in the delivery of healthcare by organizations. It expands on work done by the Office of Minority Health National Standards for Culturally and Linguistically Appropriate Services.
      www.hrsa.gov/CulturalCompetence/healthdlvr.pdf

Cultural Competence Self-Assessment Questionnaire: A Manual for Users developed by James Mason at Portland State University focuses on the cultural competence of those working with and evaluating children with disabilities and their families. The tool reviews four areas: attitude, practice, policy and structure. The appendix includes questionnaires for direct service providers and administrators. Other areas included in the assessment include: knowledge of communities, personal involvement; resources and linkages; staffing; service deliver and practice; organizational policy and procedures and reaching out to communities.
      www.eric.ed.gov/?id=ED399684

Standards of Care for Culturally Competent Nursing Care: 2011 [104]

Standard 1: Social justice	Professional nurses shall promote social justice for all. The applied principles of social justice guide nurses' decisions related to the patient, family, community, and other health care professionals. Nurses will develop leadership skills to advocate for socially just policies.
Standard 2: Critical reflection	Nurses shall engage in critical reflection of their own values, beliefs, and cultural heritage to have an awareness of how these qualities and issues can affect culturally congruent nursing care.
Standard 3: Knowledge of cultures	Nurses shall gain an understanding of the perspectives, traditions, values, practices, and family systems of culturally diverse individuals, families, communities, and populations they care for, as well as a knowledge of the complex variables that affect the achievement of health and well-being.
Standard 4: Culturally competent practice	Nurses shall use cross-cultural knowledge and culturally sensitive skills in implementing culturally congruent nursing care.
Standard 5: Cultural competence in health care systems and organizations	Health care organizations should provide the structure and resources necessary to evaluate and meet the cultural and language needs of their diverse clients.
Standard 6: Patient advocacy and empowerment	Nurses shall recognize the effect of health care policies, delivery systems, and resources on their patient populations and shall empower and advocate for their patients as indicated. Nurses shall advocate for the inclusion of their patient's cultural beliefs and practices in all dimensions of their health care.

Standard 7: Multicultural workforce	Nurses shall actively engage in the effort to ensure a multicultural workforce in health care settings. One measure to achieve a multicultural workforce is through strengthening of recruitment and retention effort in the hospital and academic setting.
Standard 8: Education and training in culturally competent car	Nurses shall be educationally prepared to promote and provide culturally congruent health care. Knowledge and skills necessary for assuring that nursing care is culturally congruent shall be included in global health care agendas that mandate formal education and clinical training, as well as required ongoing, continuing education for all practicing nurses.
Standard 9: Cross-cultural communication	Nurses shall use culturally competent verbal and nonverbal communication skills to identify client's values, beliefs, practices, perceptions, and unique health care needs.
Standard 10: Cross-cultural leadership	Nurses shall have the ability to influence individuals, groups, and systems to achieve outcomes of culturally competent care for diverse populations.
Standard 11: Policy development	Nurses shall have the knowledge and skills to work with public and private organizations, professional associations, and communities to establish policies and standards for comprehensive implementation and evaluation of culturally competent care.
Standard 12: Evidence-based practice and research	Nurses shall base their practice on interventions that have been systematically tested and shown to be the most effective for the culturally diverse populations that they serve. In areas where there is a lack of evidence of efficacy, nurse researchers shall investigate and test interventions that may be the most effective in reducing the disparities in health outcomes.

National Standards on Culturally & Linguistically Appropriate Services[105]

Goal: To advance health equity, improve quality and help eliminate health and health care disparities.

Purpose: The purpose of the enhanced National CLAS Standards is to provide a blueprint for health and health care organizations to implement culturally and linguistically appropriate services that will advance health equity, improve quality, and help eliminate health care disparities.

Principal Standard:
1. Provide effective, equitable, understandable, and respectful quality care and services that are responsive to diverse cultural health beliefs and practices, preferred languages, health literacy, and other communication needs.

Governance, Leadership and Workforce:
2. Advance and sustain organizational governance and leadership that promotes CLAS and health equity through policy, practices, and allocated resources.
3. Recruit, promote, and support a culturally and linguistically diverse governance, leadership, and workforce that are responsive to the population in the service area.
4. Educate and train governance, leadership, and workforce in culturally and linguistically appropriate policies and practices on an ongoing basis.

Communication and Language Assistance
5. Offer language assistance to individuals who have limited English proficiency and/or other communication needs, at no cost to them, to facilitate timely access to all health care and services.
6. Inform all individuals of the availability of language assistance services clearly and in their preferred language, verbally and in writing.
7. Ensure the competence of individuals providing language assistance, recognizing that the use of untrained individuals and/or minors as interpreters should be avoided.
8. Provide easy-to-understand print and multimedia materials and signage in the languages commonly used by the populations in the service area.

Engagement, Continuous Improvement, and Accountability
9. Establish culturally and linguistically appropriate goals, policies, and management accountability, and infuse them throughout the organization's planning and operations.
10. Conduct ongoing assessments of the organization's CLAS-related activities and integrate CLAS-related measures into measurement and continuous quality improvement activities.
11. Collect and maintain accurate and reliable demographic data to monitor and evaluate the impact of CLAS on health equity and outcomes and to inform service delivery.
12. Conduct regular assessments of community health assets and needs and use the results to plan and implement services that respond to the cultural and linguistic diversity of populations in the service area.
13. Partner with the community to design, implement, and evaluate policies, practices, and services to ensure cultural and linguistic appropriateness.
14. Create conflict and grievance resolution processes that are culturally and linguistically appropriate to identify, prevent, and resolve conflicts or complaints.
15. Communicate the organization's progress in implementing and sustaining CLAS to all stakeholders, constituents, and the general public.

Cultural Awareness Education *Meet the Standards	The Joint Commission	Magnet Recognition Program	Cultural & Linguistic Appropriate Standards	Utilization Review Accreditation Commission
Seminar Elements	Standard & Element of Performance (EP)	Criteria for Nursing Excellence	Standards	Core Standards
Cultural Beliefs & Values; Family	RI.01.01.01 EP#6 IM.6.20 EP#1	SE5; NK1, 7 EP 26, 29; 35	Standard 1, 7, 8	RI 2; CES 14, 17; CM 12
Health Beliefs & Practices	RI.01.01.01 EP#6 PC.01.02.01 EP#6	SE5; EP 35 NK1, 7	Standard 1	RI2; CES14, CM12
Communication Interpreters	PC.02.03.01 EP#1 RI.2.100 EP #1,2,3,4		Standard 1, 4, 5, 6, 7	CES 14, 17 Core 34, 35
Workplace Leadership Diversity	HR.01.04.01 EP#5 LD.3.20 & 3.70 EP#1,2,3 HR.2.10 & 2.30 EP#1,2,3 LD.3.120 EP#2	SE5; SE7; SE13 EP19, 20, 22, 25, NK1; 4; TL1; TL 10	Standard 2, 3, 8, 9,10, 12	Core 16; CM 8; P-NM 1 CES 18
Mental Illness	PC.01.02.11 EP#5 PC.01.02.13 EP#3		Standard 11	
Religion/ Spirituality End of Life	RI.01.01.01 EP#9 PC.02.02.13 EP#1 PC.01.02.01 EP#4		Standard 1	
Health Education Literacy	PC.02.03.01 EP#1: PC.6.10 EP#2	SE5,SE7; SE13	Standard 1,4,5, 7	CES 13; 14 , 17

Template for Cultural Awareness & Competence Seminar

Topic	Objectives	Content	Activity/Exercise
Overview	1. Discuss significance of cultural awareness & competence 2. Identify purpose of the Reflection from Common Ground Model	Elements of Reflection from Common Ground 1. Cultural Values & Beliefs 2. Education 3. Socioeconomic 4. Communication 5. Family 6. Health Beliefs & Practices 7. Religion & Spirituality	Video Social activity
History	1. Discover how one's history influences health decisions 2. Discuss historical legislative acts that promoted racism and discrimination	1. Review history or various groups and the access to health care 2. Identify reasons for & impact of legislation	Reflective exercise & small group
Demographics	1. Analyze demographic trends 2. Compare and contrast health staff & general population	1. Review demographic changes over past 100, 50 and 25 years for general population 2. Review current demographic trends for those entering the health care field	Reflective & individual

Barriers - Real & Perceived	1. Identify various socioeconomic and educational barriers 2. Discuss impact on health outcomes for diverse populations	1. Review poverty levels of various ethnic groups 2. Access to care - what are the barriers - real & perceived. 3. Level of education and the ability to navigate the system	Small group discussion then sharing with larger group
Cultural Beliefs & Values	1. Discuss the premise and goal of Culture Care Theory 2. Identify key elements of the Sunrise Model	Elements of Sunrise Model 1. Worldview 2. Cultural & Social Structure Dimensions 3. Influences 4. Transcultural Care Decisions & Actions	Reflective exercise & small group share
Communication	1. Compare and contrast meanings and style of communication for various ethnic groups 2. Neurolinguistic Programming 3. Distinguish time orientation and influence on acceptance of treatment plan	Components of communication 1. Verbal/Non Verbal 2. Tone, Pitch, Quality, Speed 3. Eye contact, Silence, Touch Time Orientation 1. Past, Present, Future 2. Plan of care goal setting format	Communication: Interactive - Pair share Read from a fictional book Time Orientation: Individual then Large group visual

Health Beliefs & Practices	1. Discuss various approaches to health, illness and treatment options	Approaches to Healthcare 1. Personalistic, Naturalistic & Biomedicine 2. Healers 3. Home remedies 4. Response to pain 5. Beliefs about mental illness and treatment	Reflective Small group discussion Small group project
Developing Plan of Care	1. Identify components for planning care	1. Acknowledge & Affirm 2. Discuss & Adjust 3. Collaborate & Change Anew	Video - Large group Reflection - Plan of Care - Small group
Religion	1. Differentiate religion from spirituality 2. Identify prayer modality and religious healing modes 3. List dietary restrictions	1. Review of spiritual leader & various religions 2. Discuss incorporation into plan of care 3. Visits by faith community	Small group discussion
End of Life	1. Compare & contrast beliefs about death 2. Discuss family involvement 3. Examine the reason for a decision to die at home or in hospital 4. Discuss the beliefs about organ donation/ transplant	1. Advanced Directives 2. Cultural beliefs about information sharing 3. Cultural beliefs about hospice 4. Beliefs about organ donation, transplant & autopsy	Small group Discussion Video Individual reflection

Health Education Patient	1. Review cultural ways of learning 2. Identify key components for a culturally accurate health education pamphlet	1. Current health education pamphlets at facility 2. Health education approaches at facility 3. Key elements of a culturally sensitive/ informative health education pamphlet	Develop a healthcare brochure that reflects the culture and language of the population
Generational	1. Identify four groups 2. List cultural beliefs/values 3. Compare and contrast the preference for communication	Generational Groups 1. Matures 2. Boomers 3. Generation X 4. Millinels Cultural Values 1. Influence of history 2. Workplace perspective Communication preference	Case presentation Large group discussion Video
Pregnancy	1. Discuss cultural & health beliefs about prenatal, intrapartum and postpartum periods	1. Pregnancy - scheduling visit 2. Hot/Cold beliefs; impact on health of mother &child during labor & postpartum 3. Beliefs about breast milk & initiation of breast feeding 4. Postpartum: length of time; purpose; roles &responsibilities	Small group discussion Video

Glossary

Acculturation: adaption of a person from one cultural group to another; may occur in stages over a long period of time

Achtgewwe: Amish term which means in order to serve, one must become aware of another's needs and then act by doing things to help.

Acupuncture: Chinese method of restoration of Yin/Yang through the use of inserting needles into meridians to remove blockage of Qi

Ahimsa: teaching of non-violence

Allopathic: health beliefs based on scientific model; technology, prescribed meds; immunizations

Amae: a term in the Japanese culture that refers to the reliance on the benevolence of another

Amulet: an object that is thought to offer protection against illness or evil spirits; tying string to wrist (Hmong), attaching safety pin to clothing (pregnant Mexican American woman)

Anghos: a Greek word a patient may use to describe a sense of choking as having a noose around one's neck

Ayurveda: ancient system of healing that includes herbal medicine, detoxification, change in lifestyle and nutrition to restore balance and health.

Bible: the holy book of Christianity

Biomedicine: an approach to health and illness; based on scientific information; cause and effect; also known as Western medicine.

Bisexual: a person whose sexual and romantic attraction is to both sexes

Botanicas: stores that provide herbs, potions, religious articles and other healing remedies

Chae-myun: a Korean term which refers to face-saving thus protecting the dignity and self respect of the family.

Choteo: a Cuban term that describe a form of humor which is displayed as ridiculing one another or exaggerating something out of proportion

Chusok: (Korean) an annual event to honor ancestors; usually held in the autumn

Class: people having the same social or economic status.

Coining: a method of healing in which a coin is placed on the skin; when dark ecchymotic spots appear it means the treatment is working.

Complicated grief: a sense of loss that includes a person being frozen or stuck in a state of chronic mourning and unable to make adaptations to life.

Curandero: healer in Mexican culture

Culture: values, beliefs, attitudes transmitted from one generation to another, often tacitly; each influence the way one sees the world

Cultural awareness: understanding one's own beliefs and values; recognizing the similarities and differences with other groups.

Cultural competence: self-awareness coupled with the knowledge of the cultural beliefs and health practices of other groups, acknowledging differences and finding common ground; providing health care that is within the cultural context of the patient.
Cultural humility: ongoing process of self-reflection and self-critique of interactions with others
Cultural imposition: imposing one's cultural views and biases on another
Cupping: applying small heated cupcake forms to skin that causes suction, thus leaving ecchymotic spots; remedy for joint and muscle pain and to remove excess wind
Disability as defined by the ADA: a physical or mental impairment that substantially limits one or more major life activities.
Discrimination: prejudicial behavior or treatment toward individuals or groups of people that involves restricting members of one group from opportunities that are available to other groups
Doshas: (in Ayurvedic medicine) includes three elements - data, pitta, and kapha which circulate in the body and regulates physiological activity
Drabarni: healer in the Roma culture
Doudy house: small house on the Amish farm where grandparents reside
Emigrate: leaves one's country to live permanently in another country

Entyo: Japanese cultural value of non-assertiveness which reflects politeness and self-restraint
Espiritismo: a religious/spiritual practice that includes both Yoruba and Catholic beliefs
Ethnicity: groups who have different experiences and backgrounds – customs, social factors, religion
Ethnocentrism: belief that one (group) is superior to another
Familimso: connotes loyalty and responsibility to family members; family first
Gay: an attraction and/or behavior which focuses on someone from the same sex or gender identity
Gender identity: a person's sense of being a woman, man or other gender, gender neutral
Gosei: fifth generation Japanese
Health care disparity: difference in the incidence, prevalence, mortality, and other adverse health conditions that exist among specific groups
Heterosexual: person who's sexual and romantic attraction is to the opposite sex or gender identity
Hilot: healer in the Filipino culture
Holistic: viewing the individual within the context of mind, body, spirit, and community
Homeopathic: a natural approach to healing
Immigrant: a person who voluntarily came to a host country

Institutional discrimination: embedded in the culture of the organization and leads to an intangible sense of prejudice - i.e. advancement, wages, contracts.
Issei: first generation Japanese
Jip-an: a term in the Korean culture that literally mean "within the house" identifies family membership, values, and traditions practiced within a particular family.
Kahuna: Hawaiian healer
Ka-moon: a term in the Korean culture that literally means "the family gate" and refers to a family's standing in the community
Karma: a key element that centers on the law of behavior and consequence
Kibun: a term in Korean culture that exemplifies ways in which harmony is achieved.
Kofte: a Greek word that refers to a form of cupping
Lesbian: refers to female same sex attraction
Literacy: the ability to read and write
Locus of control: internal is when the person believes he or she has control over their body and environment; external is the belief that anything that happens is a result of fate, luck, chance or God's will.
Magioreligious: folk medicine taking into consideration religion and folk beliefs
Marianismo: a term in the Puerto Rican culture that describes a mother's attributes which reflects the high regard for the Virgin Mary

Matiasma (or Vaskania): the Greek word for evil eye and thought of as a result of excessive admiration or envy from another person
Marielitos: the name given to the people leaving Cuba
Medicine wheel: a symbol used in the Native American culture to show wholeness by balance of mental, emotional, physical and spiritual components.
Meridians: sites where Qi flow crosses; acupuncture needles are inserted at these sites to restore flow
Moxibustion: Chinese method of healing through the use of heat
Mundang: a healer in the Korean culture
Naturalistic: an approach to health and illness; belief that illness is caused by an imbalance in the body – hot/cold, Yin/Yang, wind
Nisei: second generation Japanese
Ordnung: rules and regulations that provide standards for living the Amish life
Orisha: gods and spirits found in the Santeria
Partner: a persons' significant other exclusive of gender
Personalistic: an approach to health and illness; belief that illness is caused by intervention of a supernatural being (diety/god), nonhuman (ancestor, ghost), or human (witch, sorcerer)
Personalismo: maintain a respectful relationship
Philotimo: a Greek word that connotes the core values of honor and respect, and

reflects the obligation of each person to preserve personal and family honor.
Qi (chi): a term for energy found in all living things
Queer: a term that previously had been considered derisive and has been reintroduced as an umbrella term to identify gay, lesbian, transgender, bisexual or any sexual anatomy or gender identity
Race: a group with biological similarities
Racism: belief that one's race is superior to another
Reiki: healing method; reduces stress and restores health by transferring energy from the practitioner's hand to the client's body without touch
Religion: an organized system of beliefs; offers guidelines for practices and assurance gained through prayer and worship
Rodina: refers to the Motherland Russia
Sansei: third generation Japanese
Santeria: may be referred to as a religious/spiritual practice that includes both Yoruba and Catholic beliefs
Santero: considered a priest and traditional healer
Sexual orientation: referring to a person's physical and/or emotional attraction to the same and/or opposite sex
Shaman: healer
Simpatico: maintain smooth relationships; avoid conflict
Spirituality: a personal approach to finding life's purpose, finding meaning to life

Stenochoria: a Greek word in which patients describe a feeling of being squeezed into a narrow space
Sweat lodge: a structure that is used for healing and purification; hot rocks are placed strategically; herbs such as sweetgrass, sage, and cedar are used (Native American)
Talisman: blessed religious object that offers protection from illness and evil spirits
Torah: holy book of Judaism
Toska: suffering, considered a part of Russian life, is thought to have redemptive values
Transgender: a person whose birth identification differs from self-gender identification or gender expression
Transexual: a medical term that applies to those seeking medical/surgical treatment to live as a member of a sex category that is different than birth sex identification
Txiv Neb: healer in the Hmong culture
Varostostehos: a Greek word a patient may use to describe feeling a weight on one's chest
Vrata: a Hindu ritual that provides personal protection and blessing
Yansei: fourth generation Japanese
Yin & Yang: Chinese concept of the understanding of balance in the universe; Yin (female) and Yang (male) co-exist to ensure the complementary balance
Yoga: a physical exercise and meditative activity that helps with balance
Znahari (or Babki - old women): healers

Index

Acculturation	
Definition	56
Adjustment options	219
Obstacles (Russian)	188
Acupuncture	89
Alcoholism	
Rates	265
Consumption	265
CAGE	137
	271
Americans with Disability Act	101
2008 Amendment	102
American Sign language	104
Amish	
History	146
Beliefs/values	147
Family/Community	148
Communication	149
Health practices	149
Religion	150
Achtgewwe	149
Educational material	151
Anghos	225
Autism	172
Ayurveda	165
Bias	
Definition	34
Steps to overcome	37
Biomedicine approach	82
Body Mass Index	235
Botanicas	242
	256
Burns - Children - Amish	146
Coining	88
Communication	
High context	223
Low context	223
Culture	65
Culture of Inclusion	294
Promoting	299
Tools	302
Cultural Assessment	63
Beliefs/values	64
Communication	68
Education	73
Family	71
Healthcare practices	74
Religion/Spirituality	72
Socioeconomics	74
Space	70
Time orientation	69
Planning care	75
Cultural awareness	64
Cultural bias	33
Cultural competence	66

Cultural humility	65	Korean		174
		Languages spoken		51
Cultural imposition	33	At home (Korean)		177
		LGBT population		130
Cultural belief/value	64	Obesity		235
		Prison population		249
Cuban		Puerto Rican		251
History	237	Registered nurses		24
Beliefs/values	238	Russian		188
Family	240	Physicians		24
Communication	239	Social workers		25
Health practices	242	Socioeconomics		
Religion	241	Poverty		46
Cupping		Health Insurance		47
Definition	88	Suicide		201
Greek	225	Diabetes		
		Definition		186
		Statistics		186
Deaf		Discrimination		33
Definition	99	Institutional		296
ADA History	101			
Barriers	103	Dosha		164
Beliefs/values	104			
Family	105	Ethnicity		33
Communication	104			
Health practices	106			
Emergency preparedness	108	End of life		
Demographics		Self Determination Act		159
Census				
History	19	Entyo		206
Categories	21			
Current population	20	Espiritista		258
Current immigrants	22			
Amish	146	Ethnocentrism		33
Cuban	237			
Deaf/Hard of Hearing	100	Ethnorelativism		38
Gangs	281			
Homeless youth	115	Executive order 13583		292
Hindu	161			
Irish	267	Familioso		
Japanese	204	Definition		240

Cuban	240	Forced migration	10
Puerto Rican	252	Forced immigration	10
		Recent history	11
Gang		Healthcare reform	44
History	280		
Member category	281	Homeless youth	
		Barriers	116
Beliefs/Values	283	Beliefs/values	117
Profile	284	Communication	118
Family	285	Health care	119
		Postcards from the Edge	121
Health risk/intervention	286		
		Hot/Cold Theory	85
Greek		Irish	
History	219	History	266
Beliefs/values	220	Beliefs/values	267
Family	221	Family	270
Communication	222	Communication	268
Health practices	224	Health practices	271
Religion	226	Religion	273
Health Traditions Model	80	Japanese	
		History	203
Healers	92	Generations	203
Baba Jyotshis (Hindu)	166		213
Mundang (Korean)	179	Beliefs/values	204
Znahari (Russian)	192	Family	207
		Communication	205
Healthcare reform	44	Health practices	209
		Religion	210
Herbal therapy	91		
		Jip-an	175
Hindu			
History	161	Ka-moon	176
Beliefs/values	162		
Family	162	Karma	164
Communication	163		
Health practices	164	Kibun	177
Religion - Vedas	160		
End of life	166	Kodomo no tume ni	208
History - influence on care			
Emigration	7		

Korean		
History	173	
Barriers	174	
Beliefs/values	174	
Family	175	
Communication	177	
Health practices	179	
Religion	180	

Lesbian community
    History   129
    Definitions   130
    Health disparities   131
    Preventative screening   137
    A Welcome Environment 135
    Standards & Policies   132

Literacy
    Definition   53
    Levels   54

Locus of control   84

Marianismo   253

Matiasma   224

Naturalistic approach   84

Neurolinguistic Programming   55
    297

Obesity   235

Ordung   147

Orishas   242
    256

Personalistic approach   83

Perez-Firmat   238

Personalismo   238
    254

Philotima   220

Prejudice   33

Plan of Care   75
    Acknowledge/Affirm
    Discuss/Adjust
    Collaborate/Change

Prison
    History of Health Care   249
    Beliefs/values   252
    Communication   254
    Time Orientation   255

Puerto Rican
    History   250
    Beliefs/values   252
    Family   252
    Communication   254
    Health practices   255
    Religion   258

Qi   89
    209

Race   33

Racism   33

Reflections From Common Ground Model   67

Reiki   90

Rodina   187

Russian
- History 187
- Beliefs/values 189
- Family 190
- Communication 189
- Health practices 191
- Diabetes education 193

Santero/Saneria 242
256

SCARF Model 298

Simpatica 238
254

Shame
- Japanese 206
- Korean 178
- Russian 187
- Puerto Rican 254

Standards - Care & Practice
- Joint Commission 318
- CLAS 317
- Magnet Recognition 318
- Cultural Competence 315

Stenochoria 224

Stereotyping 34

Sweat lodge 89

Suicide
- Definition 213
- Predictors 202
- Suicide attempt 213
- Suicide Ideation 213

Toksa 191

Wind Theory 87

Varostostethos 224

Yin/Yang Theory 88

Further Reflections from Common Ground
Footnote

1. *Over 90 million Indians living on 400 million acres* . . . Charles Mann (2005). 1491: New Revelations about Americas before Columbus. New York: Random House

2. *It is frequently said that if an American Indian became a physician, he must not be 'traditional"* . . . . Still, O., Hodgins, D. (2003). Navajo Indians. In L.D. Purnell, B.J. Plankas (Eds.). Transcultural Health care: A culturally competent approach. Philadelphia: F.A. Davis

3. . . . *"the view of things in which one's own group is the center of everything."* Capell, J., Dean, E., Veenstra, G. (2008). The relationship between cultural competence and ethnocentrism of health care professionals. *Journal of Transcultural Nursing.* (19)2; 121-125.

4. "My language is me. It is an extension of mu being, my essence." Gay, G. (2004). Culturally responsive teaching: Theory, Research & Practice. New York: Teachers College Press

5. *Heritage consistency . . "is a means of identification with a traditional ethnocultural heritage."* Spector, R. (2004). Cultural diversity in health and illness. (6th Ed.). New Jersey: Pearson/Prentice Hall.

6. . . . *biomedicine, personalistic and naturalistic.* Foster, G.M. (1978). Medical Anthropology. New York: John Wiley & Sons.

7. . . . a three month old Hmong child becomes ill after her sister slams a door. Fadiman, A. (1997). The spirit catches you and you fall down. New York: Parrar, Strauss and Giroux

8. . . . *conditions that would benefit from adjunct therapy.* U.S Department of Health & Human Services. (1997). National Institute of Health: Consensus Development Program. www.consensus.nih.gov

9. *Culturally Deaf are those who a deafened pre-linguistically. . .* " Sutton, V. (2013). Physical versus Cultural Deafness: Different languages mold different cultures. Retrieved November 3, 2014 from www.signwriting.org

10. *Age . . . Population . . . Percent.* Galluadet Research Institute. (2014). About American Deaf Culture. www.gallaudet.edu

11. *Almost 44% of Deaf students do not graduate from high school.* Matthews, J.L., Parkhill, A.L., Schlehofer, D.A., Starr, M.J., Barnett, S. (2011). Role-reversal exercise with Deaf Strong Hospital to teach communication competency and cultural awareness. American Journal of Pharmaceutical Education. 75(3). pp. 1-10.

Further Reflections from Common Ground

12. *Impairment . . . Major Life Activities.* U.S. Department of Labor. (2008). Accommodation and Compliance Series: The ADA Amendments Act of 2008. Office of Disability Employment policy. Retrieved November 3, 2014 from www.eeoc.gov/laws/statutes/adaaainfo.cfm

13. *Even those who use ASL effectively may be limited by a sixth grade education.* Neuhauser, L., Ivey, S.L., Huang, D, Engelman, A., Tseng, W., Dahrouge, D., Gurung, S., Kealey, M. (2013). Availability and readability of emergency preparedness materials for Deaf and hard-of-hearing and older adult population: Issues and assessments. PLOS/ONE. 8(2). pp. 55614-55625

14. *. . . deafness is an ethnicity.* Lane, H., Pillard, R.C., Helberg,U. (2011). People of the Eye: Deaf Ethnicity and Ancestry. New York: Oxford University Press

15. *. . . It's a visual idiom, a language of the eye."* Goldberg, S. (2011). Can you see me now? Meet deaf American – a culture, a class, and a choice. *The Smart Set.* 5:14-15.

16. *The sounds on the lips may look the same as other words.* Hoag, L., LaHousse, S.F., Nakaji, M.C., Sadler, G.R. (2010). Assessing deaf cultural competency of physicians and medical students. Journal of Cancer Education. 26:175-182.

17. *. . . "physically deaf" but "culturally hearing" . . .* Sutton, V. (2013). Physical versus Cultural Deafness: Different languages mold different cultures. Retrieved November 3, 2014 from www.signwriting.org

18. *. . . effective training – The Deaf Strong Hospital Program.* Matthews, J.L., Parkhill, A.L., Schlehofer, D.A., Starr, M.J., Barnett, S. (2011). Role-reversal exercise with Deaf Strong Hospital to teach communication competency and cultural awareness. American Journal of Pharmaceutical Education. 75(3). pp. 1-10.

19. One in seven young people between the ages of 10 & 18 will run away . . National Conference of State Legislatures. (2010). Homeless and runaway youth. www.ncsi.org/issues-research/human-services/homeless-and-runaway=yout.aspx.

20. *Socialization with other homeless in the area assures economic survival. . .* Busen, N., Engebretson, J.C. (2007). Facilitating risk reduction among homeless and street-involved youth. *Journal of the American Academy of Nurse Practitioners.* 20:567-575.

21. *. . . on any given night there are 1.3 million youth living unsupervised.* National Runaway Switchboard. (2013). www.1800runaway.org

22. *Dissatisfaction with care may lead to noncompliance resulting in hospitalization or death.* National Coalition for Homeless Youth. (2008). www.nationalhomeless.org

Further Reflections from Common Ground

23. ... *Shut up and listen* ... Ensign, J., Panke, E. (2002) Young homeless women encountered physical and individual barriers in obtaining health care. *Evidence-Based Nursing.* 5(14). p. 171.

24. ... *Shut up and listen* ... Ensign, J., Panke, E. (2002) Young homeless women encountered physical and individual barriers in obtaining health care. *Evidence-Based Nursing.* 5(14). p. 171.

25. .. *Be nonjudgemental* ... Schneir, A., Stefanidis, N., Mounier, C., Ballin, D., Gailey, D., Carmichael, H. Battle, T. (2007). Trauma among homeless youth. *National Child Traumatic Stress Network.* www.nctsn.org

26. *Postcards from the Edge* ... Muir-Cochrane, E., Oster, C., Drummond, A., Fereday, J., Darbyshire, P. (2010). Postcards from the Edge: Collaborating with young homeless people to develop targeted mental health messages and translate research into practice. *Advances in Mental Health.* 9(2). pp.138-147.

27. *Lesbians have five times the risk for anxiety disorder and depression* ... Rutherford, K., McIntyre, J., Daley, A., Ross, L.E. (2012). Development of expertise in mental health service provision for lesbian, gay, bisexual and transgender communities. *Medical Education.* 46:903-913

28. ... *the result of marginalization that leads to* ... Bjorkman, M., Malterud, K. (2009). Lesbian women's experience with health care: A qualitative study. *Scandinavian Journal of Primary Health Care.* 27:238-243.

29. *Pervasive health related issues faced by lesbians* ... Substance Abuse and Mental Health Services Administration. (2012). *Top Health Issues for LGBT Populations Information & Resource Kit.* HHS Publication No. (SMA) 12-4684. Rockville, MD: Substance Abuse and Mental Health Services Administration.

30. *Do you see yourself as* ... Bradford, J.B., Cahill, S., Grasso, C., Makadon, H.J. (2014). How to gather data on sexual orientation and gender identity in clinical settings. *The Fenway Institute.* Retrieved on September 14, 2014 from www.fenwayinstitute.org.

31. ... *found the human papilloma virus in almost 30% of the women* ... Spinks, V.S., Andrews, J., Boyle, J.C. (2000). Providing health care for lesbian clients. *Journal of Transcultural Nursing.* 11(2). pp. 137-143.

32. *Recommendations for health care providers* .... Bjorkman, M., Malterud, K. (2009). Lesbian women's experience with health care: A qualitative study. *Scandinavian Journal of Primary Health Care.* 27:238-243.

Further Reflections from Common Ground

33. ... *more likely to be on a ventilator* ... Rieman, M.T., Hunley, M., Woeste, L., Kagan, R.J. (2008). Is there an increased risk of burns to Amish children? *Journal of Burn Care & Research.* 29(5). pp. 742-749.

34. ... *they saw themselves as disenfranchised from the larger community.* Wenger, F.A. Wenger, M.R. (2008). The Amish. In Purnell, L.D. (Ed.) *Transcultural Health Care: A Culturally Competent Approach.* (4th Ed.). PA: F.A. Davis.

35. ... *highlights obedience and conformity to the community's rules.* Wenger, F. (1991). The Culture Care Theory and the Ol Order Amish. In Leininger, M.M. (1991). *Culture care diversity & universality: A theory of Nursing.* New York: National League for Nursing Press.

36. *Care is expressed in the Amish term "achtgewwe"...* Wenger F.A., Wenger, M.R. (2013). The Amish. In Purnell, L.D. (Ed.) *Transcultural Health Care: A Culturally Competent Approach.* (4th Ed.). PA: F.A. Davis Company.

37. *To live simply and to care for those within the community* ... Emery, E. (1995). Amish Families. In McGoldrick, M.M., Giordano, J., Garcia-Preto, N. Ethnicity and Family Therapy. (2nd Ed.). The Guilford Press: New York.

38. *The surprise finding*... Sharpnack, P.A., Griffin, M.T., Benders, A.M., Fitzpatrick, J.J. (2010). Spiritual and alternative healthcare practices of the Amish. *Holistic Nursing Practice.* 24(2). pp. 64-72.

39. *There are over 2.5 million practicing Hindus in the United States.* Rambachan, A. (2015). The future of Hinduism in America's changing religious landscape. Huffington Post

40. *Both practices attribute good health to balance in mind, body, spirit and environment.* Miller, S.W., Lass, K.A. (2013). East Indian Hindu Americans. In Giger, J.N. (Ed.). *Transcultural Nursing: Assessment & Intervention.* (6th Ed.). Elsevier: California.

41. ... *a ritual that provides personal protection and blessing.* Bhagwan, R. (2012). Glimpses of ancient Hindu spirituality: Areas for integrative therapeutic intervention. *Journal of Social Work Practice.* 26(2). pp. 233-244.

42. *Korean Americans really measure their own self-worth, and the worth of their family*... Baker, A. (2013). Working to Combat the Stigma of Autism. *The New York Times.*

Further Reflections from Common Ground

43. *It is when parents acknowledge that home remedies are ineffective* . . . Donnelly, P.L. (2001). Korean American Family Experiences of Caregiving for their Mentally Ill Adult Children: An Interpretive Inquiry. *Journal of Transcultural Nursing.* 12(4) 292-301.

44. *. . . they isolate themselves by retreating from invitations* . . . Goehner, A.L. (2013). A Generation of Autism, Coming of Age. The New York Times Health Guide

45. *. . . . this has been an important change for most Korean Americans* . . Kim, B.C. (2005). Korean Families. In McGoldrick, M., Giordano, J., Garcia-Preto, N. (Eds) *Ethnicity & Family Therapy.* (3rd Ed.). New York: Guilford Press

46. *. . . speaking Korean, eating Korean food and practicing Korean customs.* Earp, J.K. (2013). Korean Americans. In Giger, J (Ed.) *Transcultural Nursing: Assessment & Intervention.* (6th Ed.) St. Louis, MO: Mosby/Elsevier

47. *Essential values to consider* . . . Kim, B.C. (2005). Korean Families. In McGoldrick, M., Giordano, J., Garcia-Preto, N. (Eds) *Ethnicity & Family Therapy.* (3rd Ed.). New York: Guilford Press

48. *Furthermore, 46.7% do not speak English well.* U.S Department of Commerce. (2012). Bureau of the Census. Washington DC: US Government Printing Office

49. *It is thought when one pays attention to their kibun* . . . Kim, B.C. (2005). Korean Families. In McGoldrick, M., Giordano, J., Garcia-Preto, N. (Eds) *Ethnicity & Family Therapy.* (3rd Ed.). New York: Guilford Press

50. *Cure comes by providing a balance* . . . Earp, J.K. (2013). Korean Americans. In Giger, J (Ed.) *Transcultural Nursing: Assessment & Intervention.* (6th Ed.) St. Louis, MO: Mosby/Elsevier

51. *. . . Soviet law mandates* . . . Bovovoy, A., Hine, J. (2008). Managing the Unmanageable. Medical Anthropology Quarterly. 22(1). pp. 1-26.

52. *The majority are between the ages of* . . . U.S. Department of Commerce. Bureau of the Census. (2010). American Community survey. Washington DC: US Printing Office.

53. . . . Jurcik, T., Dutton, Y.E., Jurcikova, I.S., Ryder, A.G. (2013). Russians in treatment: The evidence base supporting cultural adaptions. *Journal of Clinical Psychology.* 69(7). pp. 774-791.

54. ...Jurcik, T., Dutton, Y.E., Jurcikova, I.S., Ryder, A.G. (2013). Russians in treatment: The evidence base supporting cultural adaptions. *Journal of Clinical Psychology.* 69(7). pp. 774-791.

55. *Unfortunately, they are less likely to seek professional help* . . . Alegria, M. etal (2004). Considering context, place and culture: The national Latino and Asian American study. *International Journal of Methods in Psychiatric Research.* 13(4). 208-220.

56. *Myths and Facts.* American Psychological Association. (2012). Suicide among Asian-Americans. www.apa.org

57. . . . *viewing oneself as a burden to others* . . . Wong, Y.J., Vaughan, E.L., Lui, T, Chang, T.K. (2013). Asian Americans' proportion of life in the United States and suicide ideation: The moderating effects of ethnic subgroups. *Asian American Journal of Psychology.* 5(3) 237-242.

58. *Major predictors include discrimination, sexual orientation, alcohol and drug cohesion.* Kuroki, Y., Tilley, J.L. (2012). Recursive Partitioning analysis of lifetime suicidal behaviors in Asian Americans. *Asian American Journal of Psychology.* 3(1). 17-28.

59. *The census report indicates* . . . U.S. Department of Commerce. Bureau of the Census. (2010). American Community survey. Washington DC: US Printing Office.

60. *minor and major predictors* . . . *This concept implies that when speaker identifies with the views of the listener* . . . Ishida, D., Inouye, J. (1995). Japanese Americans. In Giger, J.N., Davidhizar, R. (Eds.) *Transcultural Nursing: Assessment and Intervention.* (2nd Ed.) St Louis, MO: Mosby.

61. *Thwarted belongingness.* Wong, Y.J., Uhm, S.Y., Li, P. (2012). Asian Americans' family cohesion and suicide ideation: Moderating and mediating effects. *American Journal of Orthopsychiatry.* 82(3). p. 309-318.5

62. *The Wartime Relocation Commission* . . . Commission on Wartime Relocation and Internment of Civilians. Personal Justice Denied: Report of the Commission on Wartime Relocation and Internment of Civilians. Seattle: University of Washington Press and Washington D.C.: Civil Liberties Public Education Fund, 1997.

63. *The phrase kodomo no tume ni, for the sake of the children.* . . Shibusawa, T. (2005). Japanese Families. In M.M. McGoldrick (Ed.) Ethnicity & Family Therapy. (3rd Ed.). Guilford Press: New York.

64. . . . *may appear reserved and passiv*e. Shibusawa, T. (2005). Japanese Families. In M.M. McGoldrick (Ed.) Ethnicity & Family Therapy. (3rd Ed.). Guilford Press: New York.

Further Reflections from Common Ground

65. *A recent Pew research study found that* . . . Pew Research Center. (2012). Asian Americans: A mosaic of faiths. www.pewforum.org

66. *Terminology* . . . Suicide Prevention Resource Center, www.sprc.org.

67. *There are three contrasting assimilation paths Theodor could take* . . . Portes, A., Zhou, M. (1993). The new second generation: Segmented assimilation and its variants. American Academy of Political and Social Science 530(1), 74-96.

68. *There are three terms used to illustrate the symptoms of stress.* Papadopoulos, I. (1999). Health and illness beliefs of Greek Cypriots living in London. *Journal of Advanced Nursing.* 29(5): 1097-1104.

69. *The heated cup then draws the blood up into the glass. It is thought that* . . . Purnell, L.D., Paulanka, B.J. (2005). Guide to Culturally Competent Health Care. F.A.Davis Company: Philadelphia, PA.

70. . . . *survey indicates 34% of Cuban American females are overweight.* Marks, G., Garcia, M. Solis, J.M. (1990). Health risk behaviors of Hispanics in the United States: Findings from HHANES, 1982-84. *American Journal of Public Health.* 80:20-26.

71. . . . *obesity rate ranges from a low of* . . .U.S. Department of Health and Human Services. (2012). Overweight and obesity statistics. National Institute of Health. NIH Publication No. 04-4158.

72. *Body Mass Index (BMI) Chart for Adults.* National Institute of Health. (2013). We Can. www.nhibi.nih.gove/health/eduational/wecan

73. . . . *would call him a "one-and-a-half .* . Bernal, G., Shapiro, E. (2005). Cuban Families. In McGoldrick, M.M. Ethnicity & Family Therapy. (3rd Ed.). Guilford Press: New York.

74. . . . *there are more than 2.2 million adults confined to state and federal prison* . . . Carson, E.A. (2014). Prisoners in 2013. Bureau of Justice Statistics, National Prisoner Statistics Program. U.S. Department of Justice: Washington D

75. *Among inmates with a persistent medical problem* . . . Wilper, A.P., Woolhandler, St., Boyd, J.W., Lasser, K.E., McCormick, D., Bor, D.H., Himmelstein, D.U. (2009). The health and health care of US prisoners: Results of a nationwide study. *American Journal of Public Health.* 99(4). pp. 666-672.

Further Reflections from Common Ground

76. *Hepatitis C found in 25-40% of the prison population* . . Wilper, A.P., Woolhandler, St., Boyd, J.W., Lasser, K.E., McCormick, D., Bor, D.H., Himmelstein, D.U. (2009). The health and health care of US prisoners: Results of a nationwide study. *American Journal of Public Health.* 99(4). pp. 666-672.

77. *Research shows that Puerto Ricans have the highest rate of asthma* . . Martin, M., Beebe, J., Lopez, L., Faux, S. (2010). A qualitative exploration of asthma self-management beliefs and practices in Puerto Rican families. *Journal of Health Care for the Poor and Underserved.* 21:464-474.

78. *According to the U.S. Census Bureau* . . . U.S. Department of Commerce. Bureau of the Census. (2012). American Community survey. Washington DC: US Printing Office.

79. *In the article Prison - Nurses behind locked doors* . . . Dryden, P. (2003). Nursing behind locked doors. *Medscape Nurses.* 5(1). Hammer, C.S., Rodriguez, B.L., Lawrence, F.R., Miccio, A.W. (2007). Puerto Rican Mothers' beliefs and home literacy practices. *Language, Speech, Hearing Service School.* 38(3). pp. 216-224.

80. *They blend African, Native American and Catholic beliefs.* Hyman, R.C., Ortiz, J., Añez, L.M., Paris, M., Davidson, L. (2006). Culture and clinical practice:Recommendations for working with Puerto Ricans and other Latinas(os) in the United States. *Professional Psychology: Research and Practice.* 6:694-701.

81. *. . cite the following statistics . . .* Blackwell DL, Lucas JW, Clarke TC. (2014). Summary health statistics for U.S. adults: National Health Interview Survey, 2012. National Center for Health Statistics. Vital Health Stat 10(260).

82. *. . .among women from a all ethnic groups* . . M McGoldrick, M. (2005). Irish Families. In McGoldrick, M.M. Ethnicity & Family Therapy. (3rd. Ed.). Guilford Press: New York

83. *They broke the constraints of gender roles so ingrained* . . O'Connor, G., (2012). Breaking the Code of Silence: The Irish and Drink. www.irishamerican.com

84. *confession, forgiveness and re-incorporation into group life.* Mullen, K., Williams, R., Hunt, K. (1996) Irish descent, religion, and alcohol and tobacco use. Addiction 91(2): 243-254.

85. *Irish history includes* . . . McGoldrick, M. (2005). Irish Families. In McGoldrick, M.M. Ethnicity & Family Therapy. (3rd. Ed.). Guilford Press: New York

86. *According to the 2010 US Census Bureau* . . . U.S. Department of Commerce. Bureau of the Census. (2010). American Community survey. Washington DC: US Printing Office

Further Reflections from Common Ground

87. *Storytelling, a famous Irish tradition . . .* McGoldrick, M. (2005). Irish Families. In McGoldrick, M.M. Ethnicity & Family Therapy. (3rd. Ed.). Guilford Press: New York

88. *My Denny, Poop betty, That Kathleen . . .* McGoldrick, M. (2005). Irish Families. In McGoldrick, M.M. Ethnicity & Family Therapy. (3rd. Ed.). Guilford Press: New York

89. *. . . believing that life will break your heart one day.* McGoldrick, M. (2005). Irish Families. In McGoldrick, M.M. Ethnicity & Family Therapy. (3rd. Ed.). Guilford Press: New York

90. *Folk treatments include . . .* Rapple, B. (2010). Irish Americans. www.everyculture.com/multi/Ha-La/Irish-American

91. *Gangs provide a sense of personal empowerment. . .* Egley, A., Howell, J.C. (2013). Highlights of the 2011 National Youth Gang Survey. Washington, DC: U.S. Department of Justice. Office of Justice Programs.

92. *. . . and engaging either individually or collectively . .* National Institute of Justice (2011). What is a gang? Definitions. Washington, D.C.: U.S. Department of Justice. Office of Justice Programs.

93. *Regular gang members account for . .* Clements, P.T. (2011). Youth gangs: Reason for concern. *Journal of Forensic Nursing.* 7:105-107.

94. *. . .an attempt to regain power/control that was lost . . .* Morris, E.J., Fry-McComish, J. (2012). Hope and despair: Diverse voices of hope from urban African American adolescent gang members. *International Journal for Human Caring.* 16(4). pp. 50-57.

95. *She identifies the following values and beliefs . . .* Morris, E.J. (2012). Respect, protection, faith and love: Major care constructs identified within the subculture of urban African American adolescent gang members. *Journal of Transcultural Nursing.* 23(3). pp.262-269.

96. *. . . results highlights the values for Mexican American gangs . . .* Tapia, H.A., Kinnier, R.T., MacKinnon, D.P. (2009). A comparison between Mexican American youth who are in gangs and those who are not. *Journal of Multicultural Counseling and Development.* 37:229-239.

97. *The following may contribute to a young person's desire to join a gang.* Kelly, S.E. (2010). The psychological consequences to adolescents of exposure to gang violence in community: An integrated review of the literature. *Journal of Child and Adolescent Psychiatric Nursing.* 23(2). pp. 61-73.

98. *The focus became* . . .Morris, E.J., Fry-McComish, J. (2012). Hope and despair: Diverse voices of hope from urban African American adolescent gang members. *International Journal for Human Caring.* 16(4). pp. 50-57.

99. *The researchers posit that there is a direct correlation between* . . . Kelly, S.E., Anderson, D.G., Hall, L., Peden, A., Cerel, J. (2012). The effects of exposure to gange violence on adolescent boys' mental health. *Issues in Mental Health Nursing.* 33:80-88.

100. . . . *key elements of an inclusive environment.* . . Pless, N.M., Maak, T. (2004). Building an inclusive diversity culture: Principles, process and practice. *Journal of Business Ethics.* 54: 129-147.

101. . . . *diverse groups that include a multitude of perspectives* . . . Kirch, D.G., Nivet, M. (2013). Increasing diversity and inclusion in medical school to improve the health of all. *Journal of Healthcare Management.* 58(5). pp. 311-313.

102. . . . *the organization looses out on the contributions* . . .Tuttas, C. (2014). Perceived racial and ethnic prejudice and discrimination experiences of minority migrant nurses: A literature review. *Journal of Transcultural Nursing.* pp. 1-7.

103. *SCARF model* . . . Rock, D. (2008). SCARF: a brain-based model for collaborating with and influencing others. *NeuroLeadership Journal.* 1: 1-9.

104. *Standards for Culturally Competent Care* Douglas, M. K., Pierce, J.U., Rosenkoetter, M., Pacquiao, D., Callister, L.C., Pollara-Hattar, M. Lauderdale, J., Milstead, J., Nardi, D., Purnell, L. (2011). Standards of practice for culturally competent care: 2011 Update. *Journal of Transcultural Nursing.* 22(4) 317-333. Used with permission

105. *Culturally & Linguistically Appropriate Services* U.S. Department of Health and Human Services. (2015). The National CLAS Standards. Office of Minority Health. Retrieved July 16, 2016 from www.minorityhealth.hhs.gov/omh

About the Author

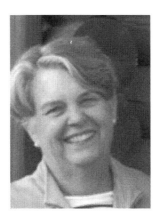

Beth Lincoln, MSN, RN

Beth Lincoln, MSN, RN received her Masters in Nursing and Women's and Family Health, with Nurse Practitioner certification from University of California, San Francisco. As a Nurse Practitioner, she has provided clinical healthcare and professional education for a diverse population, and in *Further Reflections from Common Ground*, she illustrates some of the situations in which cultural diversity may affect healthcare, including methods and means for health professionals to gain multicultural competence. Ms. Lincoln is a Certified Transcultural Nurse, credentialed by the Transcultural Nursing Society, where she currently serves as the International President. Additionally, she is an Administrator of the Intercultural Development Inventory, as certified by The Intercultural Communication Institute. Ms. Lincoln presents extensively, sharing her broad understanding and inspiring others to strive for cultural competence in providing sensitive and effective health care. Ms. Lincoln is the founder of Celemonde!, a cultural awareness educator for healthcare, scholastic and business institutions and individuals. A pathway to reflection and discovery, the Celmonde! way engages diverse professionals in a new dialogue to better appreciate how cultural issues can influence their effectiveness and decisions and create conflict in their workplace. By creating greater cultural awareness, we can open the door to common goals and better understanding. Ms. Lincoln encourages each of us to celebrate every individual as a unique opportunity to share the colorful history we all represent and the rich fabric we can become by weaving our diverse strands together.

To discover more about the Celemonde! way contact Ms. Lincoln at
www.celemonde.com

Made in the USA
Las Vegas, NV
13 December 2022

62367221R00192